Certification Exam Review for the Pharmacy Technician

Certification Exam Review for the Pharmacy Technician

Mike Johnston, CPhT

Jeff Gricar, CPhT, M.Ed
Cliff Frank, CPhT
Robin Luke, CPhT

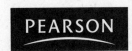

Boston   Columbus   Indianapolis   New York   San Francisco   Upper Saddle River   Amsterdam   Cape Town
Dubai   London   Madrid   Milan   Munich   Paris   Montreal   Toronto   Delhi   Mexico City   Sao Paulo
Sydney   Hong Kong   Seoul   Singapore   Taipei   Tokyo

Library of Congress Cataloging-in-Publication Data

Certification exam review for the pharmacy technician/Mike Johnston . . . [et al.].—2nd ed.
   p. ; cm.
  Rev. ed. of: The pharmacy technician series. Certification exam review. 2006.
  Includes index.
  ISBN-13: 978-0-13-510973-1
  ISBN-10: 0-13-510973-6
 1. Pharmacy technicians—Examinations, questions, etc.
I. Johnston, Mike, CPhT. II. Pharmacy technician series. Certification exam review.
  [DNLM: 1. Pharmacy—Examination Questions. 2. Pharmacists' Aides. QV 18.2 G846c 2011]
  RS122.95.J64 2011
  615'.1076—dc22

2010006188

Publisher: Julie Levin Alexander
Publisher's Assistant: Regina Bruno
Editor-in-Chief: Mark Cohen
Executive Editor: John Goucher
Development Editor: Bronwen Glowacki
Director of Marketing: Dave Gesell
Production Editor: Niraj Bhatt
Editorial Assistant: Mary Ellen Ruitenberg
Senior Marketing Manager: Harper Coles
Marketing Specialist: Michael Sirinides
Marketing Assistant: Judy Noh
Managing Production Editor: Patrick Walsh
Production Liaison: Julie Boddorf
Senior Media Editor: Amy Peltier
Media Project Manager: Lorena Cerisano

Manufacturing Manager: Ilene Sanford
Manufacturing Buyer: Pat Brown
Art Director: Christopher Weigand
Cover Designer: Christopher Weigand
Cover Images: (top left, top right, bottom right) photos.com;
  (bottom right) Getty Images
Director, Image Resource Center: Melinda Reo
Manager, Rights and Permissions: Zina Arabia
Manager, Visual Research: Beth Brenzel
Manager, Cover Visual Research and Permissions:
  Karen Sanatar
Image Permission Coordinator: Debbie Latronica
Composition: Aptara®, Inc.
Printing and Binding: Bind-Rite Graphics/Robbinsville
Cover Printer: Lehigh-Phoenix Color

Notice: The author and the publisher of this volume have taken care to make certain that the doses of drugs and schedules of treatment are correct and compatible with the standards generally accepted at the time of publication. Nevertheless, as new information becomes available, changes in treatment and in the use of drugs become necessary. The reader is advised to consult carefully the instruction and information material included in the package insert for each drug or therapeutic agent before administration. This advice is especially important when using, administering, or recommending new and infrequently used drugs. The author and publisher disclaim all responsibility for any liability, loss, injury, or damage incurred as a consequence, directly or indirectly, of the use and application of any of the contents of this volume. It is the responsibility of the reader to familiarize himself or herself with the policies and procedures set by the federal, state, and local agencies as well as the institution or agency where the reader may be employed. It is the reader's responsibility to stay informed of any new changes or recommendations made by any federal, state, and local agency as well as by his or her employing institution or agency.

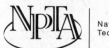

The NPTA logo is a trademark of the National Pharmacy Technician Association

The Straden-Schaden and RxPress logos are both trademarks of Straden-Schaden, Inc.

10 9 8 7 6 5 4 3

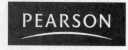

www.pearsonhighered.com

ISBN-13: 978-0-13-510973-1
ISBN-10:   0-13-510973-6

Dedication

Harry F. Banks once said, "For employee success, loyalty and integrity
are equally important as ability," which explains why I view my staff
to be so successful.
Each and every member of my team, although unique and individual,
consistently demonstrates unshakable loyalty, integrity, and incredible ability.
There is no doubt that I am blessed to work with such amazing individuals.
To each member of my team—this book is dedicated to you.

—Mike Johnston

Contents

Chapter 4
Participating in the Administration and Management of Pharmacy Practice   48

Chapter 5
Review of Pharmacy Calculations   58

Chapter 6
Pharmacy Law and Ethics   76

Preface

Certification Exam Review for the Pharmacy Technician is a core title in Pearson Education's pharmacy technician educational list of books. This text has been developed and designed to ensure greater success for the pharmacy technician student.

About the Book

More than 195,000 individuals have become nationally certified pharmacy technicians in the United States. Even though many states now require national certification to practice and more are looking to adopt such regulations, becoming certified just makes sense. Achieving recognized credentials will increase both your salary and your career opportunities.

Weighted Content

The key difference in this book is that the text content is weighted according to the national certification exam. The PTCB, the certifying board, clearly defines the percentage of content covered by the exam, yet other "review books" cover the content equally—making them, in essence, training manuals. This book has one fundamental purpose: to aid you in successfully passing the PTCB national certification exam on the first attempt. This text has removed all of the "fluff" and focuses on presenting you with the specific information and concepts you need to master to pass the exam. It is that simple.

Practice Exams

To ensure your success, we have included five complete certification practice exams. Each exam has 90 multiple-choice questions, weighted according to PTCB content guidelines, and should be completed within three hours—providing a true replica of the certification exam process.

The answers for each practice exam are provided at the back of the manual and include the rationale for each answer for the first practice exam—again, all to ensure your success!

Additional Practice

We have added three math and two trade/generic/classification tests for additional practice. Use these to improve your skills for the actual exam.

New to the Edition

In addition to enhancing and updating the original content, we have added:

- 2 additional Practice Certification Exams
- 3 brand new Math Practice Tests
- 2 Trade/Generic/Classification Practice Tests
- Student CD full of games and review material
- MyHealthProfessionsKit where students can take their practice tests in an online setting

About the Authors

Jeff Gricar, CPhT, M.Ed   Jeff Gricar earned his pharmacy technician certificate in 1986 while serving in the U.S. Navy. He has extensive work experience in institutional, retail, and home health pharmacy settings. PTCB certified for over 14 years, Jeff holds an undergraduate degree in business administration and a master's of education. A full-time faculty member since 1995, he teaches and trains pharmacy technician students in Houston Community College's ASHP-accredited Pharmacy Technician program. He is currently pursuing his doctorate degree.

Cliff Frank, CPhT   Cliff retired in 1990 from a long career in retail management and training. He then moved to Alaska with his wife and began a second career as a pharmacy technician, practicing in retail, home health care, and hospital settings. In 1998, Cliff developed a pharmacy technician training program for the University of Alaska in Anchorage, and he managed that program until 2004.

In 2003, Cliff was honored by the NPTA as the Pharmacy Technician Advocate of the Year. Today Cliff serves as the Alaska state coordinator of the NPTA and is developing a new pharmacy technician training program to be implemented across his entire home state.

Robin Luke, CPhT   Robin is a founding member of the NPTA's Executive Advisory Board, the elected body of leaders for the National Pharmacy Technician Association. She has more than 10 years of experience in institutional pharmacy, sterile product preparation, compounding, bulk manufacturing, and management, with a specialized knowledge of herbals and homeopathic treatments.

Robin has developed a variety of continuing-education programs with a strong emphasis on reducing medication errors; she also speaks at meetings and conferences across the United States.

with

Mike Johnston, CPhT   Mike is known internationally as a respected author and speaker in the field of pharmacy. He published his first book, *Rx for Success—A Career Enhancement Guide for Pharmacy Technicians*, in 2002.

In 1999, Mike founded the NPTA in Houston, Texas, and led the association from three members to more than 20,000 in less than two years. Today, as executive director of the National Pharmacy Technician Association and publisher of *Today's Technician* magazine, he spends the majority of his time meeting with and speaking to employers, manufacturers, association leaders, and elected officials on issues related to pharmacy technicians.

About the NPTA

The NPTA, the National Pharmacy Technician Association, is the world's largest professional organization established specifically for pharmacy technicians. The association is dedicated to advancing the value of pharmacy technicians and the vital roles they play in pharmaceutical care. In a society of countless associations, we believe it takes much more than a mission statement to meet the professional needs and provide the needed leadership for the pharmacy technician profession—it takes action and results.

The organization is composed of pharmacy technicians practicing in a variety of practice settings, such as retail, independent, hospital, mail-order, home care, long-term care, nuclear, military, correctional facility, formal education, training, management, and sales. The NPTA is a reflection of this diverse profession and provides unparalleled support and resources to members.

The NPTA is the foundation of the pharmacy technician profession. We have an unprecedented past, a strong presence, and a promising future. We are dedicated to improving our profession while remaining focused on our members.

For more information on the NPTA:
Call 888-247-8700
Visit www.pharmacytechnician.org

Acknowledgments

This book has been both an exhilarating and an exhausting project. To say that it is the result of a collaborative team effort would be a gross understatement.

Jeff—your revisions to this second edition have made this a better and stronger book. I appreciate your dedication to this project.

Bronwen—it has always been a pleasure working with you and I am delighted to have had you manage the revisions to the second edition. You've done a simply amazing job.

Mark—thank you for believing in my initial vision and concept for this project, which was anything but traditional. I will always remember the day we spent in New York City talking about cover concepts and the like at coffee shops and art galleries. More important, I am honored to have gotten to know you, Alex, and now little Sophie—and I consider each of you friends.

Joan—you are truly gifted at what you do. I am amazed at your ability to join this project at the point you did and to guide each daunting task into a smooth and successful accomplishment. I feel that your leadership has created a better final product.

Julie—thank you for taking risks (plural) on this project, compared with standard policies and procedures. In the end, your support and belief in this project have allowed a truly innovative product to be published.

Robin—your commitment to this project, to exceeding all expectations, and to developing the best training series for pharmacy technicians available has been amazing. You are a wonderful, gifted individual—but most important, I am thankful to call you a friend.

Andrew and Jenny—thank you supporting this project, each in your own unique ways; thank you for supporting me and the entire organization. This project tested each of us, our character, and our will, and I am honored to know you both.

Most important, I wish to thank my family. The past several years have been difficult and trying, but the strength, love, and support that you've given me have always pulled me through. Thank you.

Contributors

Andrew Cordiale, CPhT
Assistant Project Manager
Queensbury, NY

Mark Abell, PA
Lowell, FL

Jennifer Bissen, CPhT
Inteq, Inc.
Dallas, TX

Steven Hall, CPhT
NPTA
Houston, TX

Marsha Sanders, RPh
Jones County Junior College
Laurel, MS

Rhonda Wilson, CPhT
Choctaw Health Center
Philadelphia, MS

Reviewers

The reviewers of *Certification Exam Review for the Pharmacy Technician, Second Edition*, have provided many excellent suggestions and ideas for improving the text. The assistance provided by these experts is deeply appreciated.

April Cortright, CPhT
Pharmacy Technician Program Director
Sanford Brown Institute
Tampa, FL

Michael M. Hayter, Pharm D, MBA
Adjunct Instructor
Virginia Highlands Community College
Arlington, VA 24212

Janet Keleshian, CPhT
Pharmacy Technician Program Chair
CHI Institute
Broomall, PA

Mindy Koppel, CPhT
Pharmacy Technician Instructor
Pennsylvania Institute of Technology
Philadelphia, PA

Shawn McPartland, MD, JD, CPhT
Pharmacy Technician Program Chair
National College
Indianapolis, IN

Carmen Poblet, CPhT
Program Supervisor
Medix College
Smyra, GA 30080

Chris Neer, CPhT
Pharmacy Technician Lead Instructor
Remington College
Memphis, TN

Jacqueline T. Smith, RN, CPhT
Pharmacy Technician Department Director
National College
Bluefield, VA

Karen Snipe, CPhT, Med
Pharmacy Technician Program Coordinator
Trident Technical College
Charleston, SC

Bobbi Steelman, Med, CPhT
Pharmacy Technician Program Director
Daymar Colleges Group
Bowling Green, KY

Donna Stevenson, LPN, BA
Allied Health Department Chair
Remington College
Largo, FL

Getting Certified

LEARNING OBJECTIVES

After completing this chapter, you should be able to:

- Explain what a pharmacy technician is.
- Explain the different types of professional credentialing and their uses.
- List the two national pharmacy technician certification exams.
- Explain the process and reason for the creation of the Pharmacy Technician Certification Board (PTCB).
- List the categories of questioning used in the certification examination.
- Identify the score necessary to pass the Pharmacy Technician Certification Examination (PTCE).
- Explain when and how often the PTCE is offered.
- Describe the main differences between pharmacists and pharmacy technicians.
- Explain the benefits of pharmacy technician certification.
- Explain the national certification exam process.
- Explain what areas of competency are covered on the exam.
- Describe the process by which Certified Pharmacy Technicians (CPhTs) renew their certification.

Introduction

Health care in the United States is a very complicated system in which the practice of pharmacy plays an integral part. Pharmacy technicians play a valuable role in assisting pharmacists and other health care professionals as well as patients by providing ever-improving health care for U.S. citizens. In order to attain this goal, technicians need not only to be competent but also highly trained and educated. National certification for pharmacy technicians is a first step toward assuring employers, colleagues, and the public of quality health care. By becoming certified, technicians have proof of their expertise in their ever-changing field. Although certification is only a first step in gaining confidence, respect, and recognition of technicians' contribution to U.S. health care, it is a necessary and extremely important step. A technician who does not recognize the value of becoming certified is probably practicing pharmacy for the wrong reasons.

What Is a Pharmacy Technician?

The definition of a pharmacy technician is a "skilled individual, trained and educated to work in a pharmacy setting under the direct supervision of a licensed pharmacist, performing activities that do not require the professional judgment of a pharmacist." Pharmacy technicians may work in either ambulatory or institutional pharmacies.

Ambulatory pharmacies are retail or community, home health care, mail-order, clinic, or other pharmacies from which patients can obtain medications without living on site. Ambulatory pharmacies are the more numerous of the two types. *Institutional,* or *inpatient, pharmacies* are located in institutions such as hospitals, long-term-care facilities, assisted-living facilities, and retirement homes. A good rule of thumb is that if patients travel to the pharmacy or the pharmacy travels to the patient, it is an ambulatory pharmacy. If the patients and the pharmacy are housed in the same facility, it is an institutional pharmacy.

Successful pharmacy technicians are intimately involved in providing critical health care for all types of people. Therefore, pharmacy technicians must possess a wide range of knowledge and skills. They operate in strict compliance with written procedures and guidelines and answer directly to the pharmacist for the quality and accuracy of their work.

Pharmacy technicians deal with private medical and insurance information as well as with dangerous and perishable substances and must possess the highest ethical and professional standards. Breaches in this public trust can lead to serious consequences. When the one-hour-photo guy makes a mistake, you lose your pictures and he could ultimately lose his job. When a pharmacy technician makes an error, the result can be serious health consequences and even death. As their direct supervisor, the pharmacist is ultimately responsible for checking technicians' work; however, a technician can be held legally liable for errors of negligence or omission.

As one of the oldest professions, the practice of pharmacy has evolved over centuries and continues evolving to this day. The profession of pharmacy technician is more recent in its origin but is an integral part of the practice of pharmacy. Depending on the practice site, a technician may be referred to as a technologist, aide, or assistant, but the skills needed remain the same. Technicians perform more and more tasks previously reserved for pharmacists, so training, education, and certification are becoming increasingly important to the safety of the patient, in part because a mistake due to carelessness or ignorance could lead to a serious health consequence or death.

In the past, most technician training was on-the-job training (OJT). By its very nature, however, OJT is employer-provided training designed specifically for, and limited to, the tasks required in the job for which the technician is being trained. In most cases, OJT cannot provide instruction or understanding as to the theory or background surrounding pharmacy practice. For example, pharmacy technicians in all pharmacy settings routinely perform mathematical calculations. Accuracy in calculating is imperative for the safety of the patient, and that intensity of training is not often provided by OJT.

Pharmacy also has its own language that technicians must master. Prescriptions contain abbreviations, symbols, and terminology all designed to help prescribers communicate with the pharmacy while ensuring the safety and accuracy of the medications dispensed. The abbreviations BID, TID, and QID, although similar, all have different meanings and can be easily confused. The abbreviations OS and AS, if confused, could potentially cause eye damage.

Training and education are two very separate processes. We can train a monkey to answer a door when the bell rings. We cannot, however, make that monkey understand social relationships or even why he is doing what he is doing. As technician tasks and prescription volume increase, OJT simply is no longer practical in most settings. Education is the key to the success and longevity of a pharmacy technician.

What Is Certification?

Professionals are identified in different ways, all of which are useful in the proper settings. Credentialing, accreditation, registration, licensing, and certification are some of the most common. It is important to understand these terms, as there has been much confusion in the pharmacy profession over their use.

- *Credentialing* grants some kind of formal recognition of professional or technical competence.
- *Accreditation* usually refers to institutions that have met certain standards set by an agency and carry that agency's stamp of approval.
- *Registration* is simply the process of listing, or being named to a list.
- *Licensing* is permission granted by a government entity for an individual to perform an activity. The person has to meet certain standards, usually designed to protect the public.
- *Certification* is recognition granted by a nongovernmental agency that attests that an individual has met the required level of competency.

When a pharmacy technician becomes certified, the Pharmacy Technician Certification Board (PTCB) or the Institute for the Certification of Pharmacy Technicians (ICPT) verifies that the candidate has met the board's standards for skills and knowledge necessary to gain the right to use CPhT (Certified Pharmacy Technician) after his or her name. Certification indicates that the technician possesses knowledge and skills of a certain level determined by the certification agency and is a signal to employers, co-workers, and patients of a minimum level of competence.

What Is the PTCB?

In 1995, the American Pharmacists Association (APhA), the Illinois Council of Health-System Pharmacists (ICHP), the Michigan Pharmacists Association (MPA), and the American Society of Health-System Pharmacists (ASHP) came together to create the Pharmacy Technician Certification Board (PTCB). The Pharmacy Technician Certification Examination (PTCE) was then created in an effort to identify and standardize knowledge and skills necessary to be a competent pharmacy technician in all types of pharmacy sites. The PTCB is the largest national certification agency for pharmacy technicians.

The PTCB Exam Criteria

The PTCE is offered continuously throughout the year. The exam consists of 90 multiple-choice questions, which must be completed within two hours. Applications for the exam are accepted 24 hours a day; after a candidate is approved, he or she has 90 days to complete the exam. If a candidate fails the first exam, he or she may retake it up to three times. For the first two retakes, candidates are required to wait 60 days before taking the exam again. For the third retake, candidates are required to wait six months before taking the exam again. However, a pharmacy technician who receives proper guidance and who studies should only have to sit for the examination once.

The criteria used by the PTCB measure the candidate in three areas of competence:

- **Assisting the Pharmacist in Serving Patients.** This includes knowledge about assisting the pharmacist in dispensing prescriptions, distributing medications, and collecting and organizing information. These responsibilities include screening prescriptions for accuracy and validity; counting, measuring, and compounding medications; and performing insurance billing. This knowledge accounts for approximately 66% of the exam.

- **Maintaining Medication and Inventory Control Systems.** Questions in this area test knowledge about placing and receiving drug orders, storing drugs correctly, removing outdated drugs from inventory, and organizing and monitoring pharmacy supply levels. This knowledge accounts for approximately 22% of the exam.

- **Participating in the Administration and Management of Pharmacy Practice.** Questions in this area test knowledge of general pharmacy operations, including maintaining facilities, equipment, and information systems; servicing automated dispensing systems; and performing computer maintenance. This knowledge accounts for approximately 12% of the exam.

The questions on the exam are weighted, meaning that certain questions are worth more points than others, and the final score is based on the number of questions that are answered correctly. All PTCB exams are computer-based, and examinees immediately receive a "pass" or "fail" result upon completion of the exam. To pass the exam and become certified, a candidate must attain a score of at least 650 out of a possible 900 points.

Candidates must meet the following eligibility requirements in order to sit for the exam:

- High school diploma or its equivalent (e.g., a GED or foreign diploma).
- No felony conviction.
- No drug- or pharmacy-related convictions, including misdemeanors. These violations must be disclosed to the PTCB.
- No denial, suspension, revocation, or restriction of registration or licensure, consent order, or other restriction by any state Board of Pharmacy. No admission of misconduct or violation of regulations of any state Board of Pharmacy.

Complete application and eligibility requirement information can be found at www.ptcb.org.

What Is the ExCPT?

The second and lesser known of the two national exams is the Exam for the Certification of Pharmacy Technicians (ExCPT). Administered by the Institute for the Certification of Pharmacy Technicians (ICPT), the ExCPT is a standardized and psychometrically sound exam that can be taken one to two days after registering for it. A pyschometrically sound exam is designed using standards that ensure the evaluation tool provides a nonbiased, sound, and accurate representation of the examinee's knowledge. Complete application and eligibility requirement information can be found at www.nationaltechexam.org.

Why Get Certified?

Since its inception with the PTCB, national certification has become a widely recognized standard of achievement accepted by employers and fellow technicians as a sign of competence. As the role of the pharmacy technician continues to expand, encompassing mechanical and routine aspects of pharmacy practice, so does the need for technicians to work accurately and efficiently with less direct supervision. Increasingly, most retail, hospital, extended-care facility, compounding, and admixture pharmacies are requiring national certification as a condition for employment.

Although it is optional in some states, national certification is the best way to ensure the competence of a practicing pharmacy technician in terms of hireability, job security, and career advancement. Those who hire, work with, or entrust their health care to a CPhT can be assured that the technician has the skill, knowledge, and professionalism to do the job successfully, as well as a desire to continue learning and growing in the profession. A better question than "Why get certified?" is "Why not get certified?"

Recertification

As in most health care professions, CPhTs must keep their knowledge current in order to remain effective members of the health care team. Recertification helps to assure employers, colleagues, and the public that the practicing pharmacy technician has maintained a minimum level of competence and knowledge and that technicians stay current on the many changes and breakthroughs each year in the science of pharmacy.

Recertification with both PTCB and ICPT is required every two years, at which time, technicians must show proof that they have participated in 20 contact hours of approved technician education, with at least one contact hour in pharmacy law.

Continuing-education credits can come from a variety of sources. National associations, such as the National Pharmacy Technician Association (NPTA), as well as state and local chapters of the American Society of Health-System Pharmacists (ASHP) and the American Pharmacists Association (APhA) are excellent sources for continuing-education credits. Also accepted are certain accredited college credits and employer-driven continuing education.

SUMMARY

As the role of pharmacy technicians continues to expand, certification has become an integral part of assuring pharmacists, employers, and the public that an individual has achieved competency in this field. Many states now require certification as a prerequisite to work as a pharmacy technician.

CHAPTER REVIEW QUESTIONS

1. A technician who has successfully completed the national certification examination is known as a(n):
   a. RphT
   b. CPT
   c. PCT
   d. CPhT

2. The attesting that an individual has met the required levels of competency, usually granted by a nongovernmental institution, is known as:
   a. certification
   b. accreditation
   c. licensure
   d. registration
   e. credentialing

3. The PTCE is the certification exam offered by the:
   a. APhA
   b. ASHP
   c. NPTA
   d. ICPT
   e. PTCB

4. How many hours of continuing education are required for each recertification cycle?
   a. 1 hour
   b. 10 hours
   c. 15 hours
   d. 20 hours
   e. 30 hours

5. How often must certified pharmacy technicians renew their certification?
   a. every year
   b. every 2 years
   c. every 3 years
   d. every 4 years
   e. every 5 years

6. Which of the following statement(s) is/are true?
   a. The PTCB exam is computer-based.
   b. The PTCB exam is offered continuously throughout the year.
   c. The questions on the PTCB are categorized into three distinct knowledge areas.
   d. All of the above statements are true.
   e. Only a and c are true.

7. The PTCB examination consists of:
   a. 125 questions
   b. 90 questions
   c. 75 questions
   d. 100 questions

8. How much time are candidates sitting for the PTCE given to answer all the questions?
   a. 1 hour
   b. 3 hours
   c. $2\frac{1}{2}$ hours
   d. 2 hours

9. True or false: A pharmacy technician may practice only under the direct supervision and authority of a pharmacist.
   a. true
   b. false

10. True or false: At least 22% of the Pharmacy Technician Certification Examination questions deal with medication distribution and inventory control systems.
    a. true
    b. false

Assisting the Pharmacist in Serving Patients

LEARNING OBJECTIVES

After completing this chapter, you should be able to:

- List the common duties and responsibilities of a pharmacy technician.
- Define policies and procedures as they relate to the practice of pharmacy.
- Describe the differences between quality-control and quality-improvement mechanisms.
- Define a prescription or medication order and list ways by which it is received.
- List the elements of a prescription.
- Describe the formula for checking a Drug Enforcement Administration (DEA) number's authenticity, and list warning signs of a forged prescription.
- Explain the importance of maintaining patient profiles.
- Describe the most common types of reactions and interactions.
- Describe steps for proper order processing.
- List and use common sig codes used in prescription labeling.
- List the steps necessary for transferring a prescription.
- List and explain the nine guidelines for compounding medications.
- List and describe common equipment used in pharmacies.
- Describe the six critical steps in intravenous admixture preparation.
- List and describe extra precautions necessary for preparing cytotoxic medications.
- Describe the Food, Drug, and Cosmetic Act (FDCA) prescription labeling requirements.
- List regulations governing prescription refills.
- List the sources of drug information used in pharmacies.
- Describe the insurance billing process.
- List common alert messages used in insurance billing.

Introduction

Assisting the pharmacist is at the core of being a pharmacy technician. With the exception of patient counseling, receiving new prescriptions, and performing the final verification of a prescription, a pharmacy technician can do almost any task in most pharmacy practice settings. Of course, the pharmacy technician always works under the direct supervision and authority of a pharmacist. Today's quickly expanding health care industry has a great need for skilled and knowledgeable technicians who possess in-depth understanding of the prescription process as well as a working knowledge of drugs, interactions, and computer systems, among other things.

This chapter explores the many ways a pharmacy technician becomes a valuable asset to any pharmacy site and the "right hand" of a very busy pharmacist.

Duties of a Pharmacy Technician

Pharmacy technicians perform a myriad of tasks, the outcomes of which are crucial to the health and well-being of the patient. Before there were pharmacy technicians, pharmacists performed all of the tasks associated with the practice of pharmacy. Today, the main goal of the pharmacy technician is to assist the pharmacist in meeting the pharmaceutical health care needs of the patient. The following is just a sampling of the tasks commonly performed by technicians in two of the main practice settings (retail and hospital):

- Answer basic questions that do not require professional judgment, such as item location or referral to the pharmacist.
- Answer the phone.
- Check, order, receive, and restock pharmacy inventory.
- Clean and maintain pharmacy equipment.
- Compound nonsterile pharmaceuticals.
- Deliver medications to patients and other medical personnel.
- Fill medication orders.
- Inventory and restock "crash cart" medications.
- Inventory, restock, and maintain pharmacy robotics and technology.
- Operate cash registers.
- Perform pharmaceutical calculations.
- Prepare and process insurance claims.
- Prepare medications.
- Prepare prescription labels.
- Prepare sterile intravenous admixtures, including IVPB, LVP, IVP, chemotherapy, and TPN.
- Provide excellent customer service.
- Receive and process refill requests.
- Receive new prescriptions and review for completeness.

Policies, Procedures, and Technicians

Policies and procedures (P&Ps) are valuable guides for any employee, especially pharmacy technicians. All employers will have their own P&Ps, in a written or electronic manual, that must be readily and easily accessible to employees. Common policies and procedures include the following:

- Hiring requirements
- Employee benefits

- Expected employee behavior and standards
- Monitoring of patient allergies
- Management of toxic or dangerous drugs
- Procedures for protecting patients from errors
- Proper handling and distribution of drugs
- Proper handling of cytotoxic drugs
- Correct aseptic technique for compounding and admixtures
- Emergency procedures for disasters: fire, earthquake, tornado, and so on

P&Ps are not put intended to put restrictions on the pharmacy technician, but instead to give clear and precise directions that will guide the technician in proper pharmacy protocol, the safe handling of drugs, and safety protection, all of which can protect the pharmacy technicians from career-ending errors. However, if a policy or procedure is ambiguous or unclear, the pharmacy technician should always consult the pharmacist for clarification.

Quality Assurance

Quality assurance (QA) can be defined as the ongoing set of activities used to assure that the processes used in the preparation of drug products meet predetermined standards of quality. QA programs determine that facilities, systems, and written policies and procedures are adequate and are followed to assure that all final products meet the institution's requirements. You can think of QA as the *overall plan* for maintaining quality.

Quality-assurance mechanisms are divided into two important categories that should not be confused: quality control and quality improvement. Both are critical to the operation of a pharmacy, but each has its separate place in the ongoing quest to improve patient health care and safety.

Quality Control

Quality control (QC) is a process of checks and balances (or procedures) that are followed to ensure that end products meet or exceed specified standards (i.e., zero errors and zero problems). Quality control is the *day-to-day management* of quality in the pharmacy, which is necessary to prevent defective products from reaching the patient.

Quality Improvement

Quality improvement is an ongoing process that monitors, evaluates, and identifies problems by study, reports, charting, and collecting all of the pertinent information. Technicians often play a valuable role in this process by helping to collect, organize, and chart quality-improvement data.

Defining the Prescription

A *prescription* is a written, verbal, or electronic order from a practitioner, or from his or her authorized agent, to a pharmacist for a drug or drug device to be dispensed. A prescription (Rx) may be handwritten and given to the patient or health care professional for presentation to the pharmacy, may be communicated directly to the pharmacist by telephone or fax, or may be sent electronically from a practitioner's computer to the pharmacist's computer. Electronic prescriptions are accepted only if they are sent via a secure system. Verbal prescriptions can be received only by a pharmacist and should be reduced to proper written format immediately. Most noncontrolled prescriptions expire one year from the date the prescription was written by the prescriber.

A written prescription has four main parts:

- The *superscription* consists of the heading, where the symbol Rx (believed to be an abbreviation for *recipe,* Latin for "take thou") is found.

- The *inscription,* also called the body of the prescription, provides the names and quantities of the main active ingredient(s) of the prescription as well as the dose and dosage form.
- The *subscription* indicates to the pharmacy the quantity to dispense.
- The *signature* or *signa* or *sig* gives instructions to the patient on how, how much, when, and for how long the drug is to be taken.

The prescription, known as a *medication order* in an institutional pharmacy setting, is a legal document that must be treated carefully. Like any legal document, it may not be altered without the express permission of all parties involved. The pharmacist's duty is to see that this order is carried out exactly as the prescriber intended. A well-trained and educated technician is invaluable in assisting the pharmacist in filling prescriptions.

Because laws vary from state to state, it is important to be aware of all the legal regulations in your state as well as any additional requirements imposed by your employer. Regulations regarding the manner in which a prescription arrives are part of the security system set up to protect the patient, the prescriber, the pharmacist, and the technician from errors as well as fraud.

The Path of a Prescription from Prescriber to Patient

The typical path of a prescription from the time it is written by a prescriber to the time it is dispensed to the patient is as follows:

- The prescriber writes the prescription and gives it to the patient or the patient's agent.
- The patient or the patient's agent delivers the prescription to the pharmacy.
- The technician reviews the prescription for completeness and authenticity.
- The technician enters the prescription into the computer system, which includes the billing process, and a prescription label is generated. The technician verifies that the label matches the written prescription exactly.
- The technician selects the drug to be dispensed, matching the National Drug Code (NDC) on the stock bottle with the prescription label.
- The technician fills the prescription manually (by counting, measuring, or pouring) or by using an automated drug-dispensing system.
- The technician attaches the label.
- The technician presents the finished product to the pharmacist for final verification.
- The pharmacist approves the prescription for dispensing, and the completed prescription is properly stored along with any pertinent information sheets.
- The patient picks up the prescription, at which time the pharmacist offers counseling.

Reviewing Prescriptions and Medication Orders

It is imperative that the technician review each prescription and mediation order to ensure that it is complete. In a retail setting, a prescription that is not complete will cause extra waiting time for the patient, because the pharmacy will have to contact the doctor. In a hospital, an incomplete medication order means that the pharmacy will not dispense the medication to the nurse to give to the patient. Either way, the technician can be the first line of defense in ensuring that prescriptions and medication orders contain all the required information.

Required Information on a Prescription

Federal law requires all prescriptions contain certain information before the order can be filled. Be aware that state boards of pharmacy may have additional prescription information requirements. The receiving technician must ensure that the following information is included when the prescription is accepted. Never assume any information that might be missing. In cases of missing information, be sure to consult with your pharmacist.

- **Patient name.** A technician must ensure that the name is the patient's complete legal name, not a shortened name or nickname. Double-check the name while the patient is still at your pharmacy and correct any discrepancies at this time.

- **Drug name.** The name of the drug may written as a trade name, a generic name, or both. If the prescriber wants the trade-name drug dispensed, he or she will indicate "dispense as written." If the prescriber indicates "substitution permitted," then the pharmacy can substitute an equivalent generic drug for the trade-name drug prescribed.

- **Drug strength.** The drug strength indicates the potency of the drug that the pharmacy will dispense to the patient. It is important that prescribers indicate the strength of the drug they want prescribed, because many drugs are available in several different strengths. Drug strengths of solid drugs are most commonly expressed as milligrams (mg), micrograms (mcg), grams (g), or milliequivalents (mEq). Liquid drug strengths are expressed as mg, mcg, g, or mEq per a volume measurement (e.g., 5 mg/mL or 10 mEq/5 mL).

- **Dosage form.** The dosage form is the physical manifestation of the drug, such as tablet or suspension. The dosage form must be indicated because many drugs are available in several different dosage forms. The dosage form also tells technicians where in the pharmacy inventory they will find the medication. Common dosage forms include:

Tablet	Capsule
Liquid	Suspension
Elixir	Solution
Ointment	Cream
Suppository	Inhalation aerosol
Ophthalmic solution or suspension	Gelcap

- **Route of administration.** The route of administration (ROA) indicates how the drug will enter or be applied to the body. The ROA is critical especially when it comes to intravenous (IV) medication, because the same medication can be given by several different IV routes. It is important to understand that the same drug may have a different patient dose depending on the ROA. For example, ranitidine (Zantac) is given at a dose of 150 mg by mouth, but at a dose of only 50 mg intravenously. Common routes of administration include:

Oral	Intravenous
Topical	Ophthalmic
Otic	Transdermal
Inhalation	Sublingual

- **Patient dose.** The patient dose indicates how much of the medication the patient is prescribed to take each time.

- **Frequency or schedule of administration.** This tells the patient how often to take the medication. Common schedules of administration include:

Daily	BID
TID	QID
q4h	q6h
q8h	q12h

- **Quantity to dispense.** This indicates how much medication is being prescribed to the patient. The quantity may be exact (e.g., Disp: 30 caps), or the pharmacy technician may have to calculate the quantity (e.g., Disp: 30-day supply). In many states, quantities of controlled substances must be written both numerically and in words (e.g., Disp: 10 (ten) tabs).

- **Prescriber's name and signature.** If the prescription cannot be attributed to an authorized prescriber or if the prescriber does not sign the prescription manually, it cannot be filled. Many pharmacies keep an alphabetical index file with the printed name followed by a signature example for each prescriber. This provides an easy reference for newer technicians to use while learning the signatures of doctors in their area.

All the required parts of a prescription give valuable information that will ensure the right patient gets the right medication in the right strength and form at the right time. A technician cannot "fill in the blanks" or "assume" anything at any time. Part of a technician's duty is to make sure the prescriber's exact directions are followed in the selection, preparation, and administration of the patient's medication order; the technician must refer any questions to the pharmacist, who will give further directions.

Requirements for Controlled-Substance Prescriptions

All controlled substances have some potential for abuse, so prescriptions for these substances have additional requirements to make them even more difficult for abusers or forgers to obtain. Additional information required on a controlled-substance prescription includes:

- The patient's address
- The prescriber's name, address, and Drug Enforcement Administration (DEA) registration number
- Written in ink with no signs of alteration

All prescribers of controlled substances are assigned a DEA number that allows them to prescribe controlled substances, and all controlled-substance prescriptions must contain the prescriber's DEA number. Without a valid DEA number, the pharmacy is not allowed to fill the controlled-substance prescription.

A valid DEA number consists of two letters, six digits, and one check digit. The first letter indicates the type of registrant. The first letter of a prescriber's DEA number will be A, B, or F, or M if the prescriber is a mid-level practitioner such as a physician's assistant. The second letter will be the first letter of the prescriber's last name. The remaining seven digits follow a numerical formula that the technician must verify before filling a controlled-substance prescription.

To verify a DEA number:

1. Add the first, third, and fifth digits of the DEA number.
2. Add the second, fourth, and sixth digits, then multiply that sum by 2.
3. Add the two totals together; the last digit of the answer should match the last digit of the DEA number (check digit).

EXAMPLE: Dr. William Frank—DEA#:   AF1437537.

$$1 + 3 + 5 = \underline{9}$$
$$4 + 7 + 3 = 14 * 2 = \underline{28}$$
$$9 + 28 = \underline{37}$$

The final digit, 7, is a match, so this is a valid DEA number.

Scope of Practice

Each state has its own laws governing who can prescribe which types of medications. Most states give physicians wide latitude, while other health care professionals may be limited to their *scope of practice*. For example, a veterinarian may prescribe for animals but not humans. A dentist may prescribe drugs for pain or infection, but not eyedrops. In most cases, prescribers are discouraged and may be prohibited from prescribing for family members. The pharmacy technician can be of great help to a busy pharmacist by incorporating knowledge of prescribers and their practices when screening prescriptions.

In many areas, the local DEA office sends out notices periodically to warn pharmacies that certain prescribers are prohibited from prescribing certain drugs or any drugs for a given period of time. These notices should be posted in plain view of the pharmacy staff and referred to often.

Patient Profiles and Changes

Pharmacy technicians are responsible for setting up and maintaining patient profiles. These profiles, besides being confidential legal records, give the pharmacist a "complete view" of the patient. Information on a patient profile usually includes:

- **Patient demographic information**—complete name, identification number, address, phone number, date of birth, sex, parent or guardian.
- **Insurance and billing information**—insurance company name, phone number, group number, patient code, and any other information that may be needed.
- **Medical history**—any past and present medical conditions, including allergies. If a patient has allergies, the profile may also include the severity of the last reaction. Reactions are rated as 1 (nausea), 2 (rash or hives), or 3 (trouble breathing, or a reaction that requires immediate medical intervention. This information helps the pharmacist understand the possible risks of allergic reaction and plays a vital role in any possible decision to contact the prescriber. Technicians must be aware that many people believe that they have an allergy to a drug when, in reality, the drug simply upsets their stomach.
- **Prescription history**—a listing of all prescriptions that have been filled at that particular pharmacy. This may include over-the-counter (OTC) medications as well as herbal products the patient may be taking.
- **Prescription preferences**—whether the patient prefers brand-name or generic medications, or whether they want non-child-resistant, "easy-off" container closures.
- **Refusal of information**—whether the patient has ever refused to sign pharmacy documents, including HIPAA and insurance forms.

Patient profiles in hospital pharmacies may also include the patient's account number, room number, diagnosis, names of practitioners, allergies, dietary restrictions, and any language barriers or disabilities. This information then becomes part of the patient's permanent hospital medical record.

One of the most important items in a patient's profile is the name. Several challenges arise when a patient goes by a nickname or has changed name as a consequence of marriage, adoption, or divorce. To avoid dispensing a prescription to the wrong patient or adding multiple incomplete profiles for the same patient to the computer, technicians can verify that they have the correct patient by comparing the name against the date of birth and/or address and phone number in the patient profile. By performing this simple double-check, technicians can ensure that the correct prescription is being processed for the correct patient.

Technicians need to ensure that the patient's profile is always kept up to date with the correct information. When reviewing prescriptions, technicians should always ask patients if there have been any changes to their profile—especially, changes to address, phone number, or insurance carrier.

Drug Interactions

A drug interaction occurs when a substance or condition affects the pharmacologic activity of a drug. In most cases, the interaction causes an increase or decrease in the drug's effect, or sometimes a completely different, unintended effect. Most pharmacy computer systems have automatic warning systems that will alert the technician to possible adverse reactions. A qualified and competent pharmacy technician will have a working knowledge of these potential problems. It is imperative that any time the computer alerts the technician to a potential problem, reaction, or allergy, the technician immediately informs the pharmacist. It is out of the scope of practice for a technician to override most of these alerts. Some of the most common warnings/alerts include:

- **Therapeutic Duplication.** A therapeutic duplication warning is an indication that the patient has more than one active prescription for the same medication or has two different medications that produce the same or similar effect. This is common among patients who have more than one doctor writing prescriptions for them.

- **Drug–Drug Interaction.** A drug–drug interaction alert is an indication that the patient has a medication in his or her profile that will cause an unfavorable reaction if it is taken along with the new prescription. A common drug–drug interaction occurs with warfarin and aspirin.

- **Drug–Food Interactions.** A drug–food interaction indicates that the medication being prescribed interacts with certain foods.

- **Drug–Disease Interactions.** A drug–disease interaction occurs when a past, current, or present patient medical condition precludes use of the drug.

- **Drug–Lab Interactions.** In a hospital setting, certain medical tests may interfere with the patient's medications, therefore requiring temporary suspension of the patient's drug therapy.

- **IV Incompatibility.** An IV incompatibility alert indicates that there is a potential interaction if two or more IV drugs are mixed together in the same container. For instance, total parenteral nutrition (TPN) with both calcium and phosphate would trigger an alert, because mixing these substances together can cause a precipitate to form.

REMEMBER

All warnings and alerts should be forwarded to the pharmacist for further investigation and possible consultation.

Processing Prescriptions

After a technician receives a prescription, the challenge is to get the right medication to the right patient in the right form and strength at the right time, and at the same time, charge the responsible party. Although each pharmacy may differ in some aspects, there is a basic procedure for processing and filling a prescription.

1. Review the prescription or medication order to ensure that it is complete. Reviewing the prescription includes making sure the patient is in the database and collecting any changes that need to be made to the patient profile (demographic, history, insurance/billing).

2. Review the patient's profile in relation to the new order you are processing. Is the patient already on similar medications? Can this new medication react unfavorably with any other medication he may be taking? Has the patient reported any allergies that may be triggered by this medication? Although the pharmacy's software automatically checks for interactions, the main responsibility lies on the technician and ultimately the pharmacist to protect the patient and follow the prescriber's directions.

3. Select the prescribed medication in the right dosage form, strength, and quantity from the formulary database in your pharmacy's computer. The best way to choose the correct medication is to choose by the National Drug Code (NDC).

The NDC number is a ten-digit, three-segment, permanent and unique number assigned to the drug by the U.S. Food and Drug Administration (FDA) when it first becomes available in the United States.

- The first segment is called the *labeler code* and identifies the manufacturer or distributor of the drug.
- The second segment is called the *product code* and identifies the dosage form, strength, and formulation.
- The third segment is called the *package code* and identifies the type and size of the drug package.

By matching the number on the label with the number on the stock bottle, the technician is ensuring that the correct drug has been selected.

4. Next, generate the prescription label. The directions typed on the label must be exactly the same as the prescriber intended, as well as clear enough for the patient to understand and follow. These directions should answer the following questions:

- What should the patient do with the drug? (ex. Take, Apply, Insert)
- What should the patient Take, Apply, Instill? (ex. Take *one tablet,* Apply *ointment,* Instill *2 drops*)
- How should the patient Take, Apply, Insert the drug? (ex. Take one tablet *by mouth,* Apply ointment *to rash,* Instill 2 drops *in each eye*)
- How often should the patient Take, Apply, Insert the drug? (ex. Take one tablet by mouth *two times daily,* Apply ointment to rash *every 8 hours,* Instill 2 drops in each eye *4 times daily*)

Most computer systems designed for prescription dispensing use a series of sig codes. These sig codes or abbreviations are designed to save time and to standardize label language. For example, if you type, "1t po tid prnp," the label will read, "Take 1 tablet by mouth three times daily as needed for pain."

The following table lists some of the most common abbreviations/sig codes used in prescription processing.

ABBREVIATION/SIG CODE	DEFINITION
a	before
ac	before meals
ad	right ear
a.m.	morning
amp	ampoule
a.s.	left ear
a.u.	both ears or each ear
BID	two times daily
cap	capsule
cc	cubic centimeter
CHF	congestive heart failure
DW	distilled water
ECT	enteric coated tablet
fl or fld	fluid

(Continued)

ABBREVIATION/SIG CODE	DEFINITION
fl. oz	fluid ounce
GI	gastrointestinal
gr	grain
gtt	drop
gtts	drops
HA	headache
HBP	high blood pressure
h or hr	hour
HT or HTN	hypertension
IA	intra-arterial
ID	intradermal
IM	intramuscular
IV	intravenous
IVP	intravenous push
IVPB	intravenous piggyback
lb	pound
mcg or µg	microgram
mEq	milliequivalent
mg	milligram
mg/kg	milligrams per kilogram
ml or mL	milliliter
ml/hr	milliliters per hour
n&v or n/v	nausea and vomiting
NS	normal saline
NTG	nitroglycerin
od	right eye
os	left eye
ou	both eyes or each eye
p	after
pc	after meals
p.m.	evening
po	by mouth
pr	rectally
prn	as needed
q	every
q4h	every 4 hours
q6h	every 6 hours
q12h	every 12 hours
q24h	every 24 hours

ABBREVIATION/SIG CODE	DEFINITION
qd	every day
qh	every hour
QID	four times daily
qs	a sufficient quantity
sl	sublingual
SOB	shortness of breath
ss	one-half
sq or subq	subcutaneous
stat	immediately or now
supp	suppository
susp	suspension
tab	tablet
tbsp	tablespoon
TID	three times daily
ud	as directed
ung	ointment
UTI	urinary tract infection
wk	week

The following table illustrates the transcription of sig codes to complete patient directions.

SIG CODES ENTERED INTO COMPUTER BY PHARMACY TECHNICIAN	PATIENT DIRECTIONS
T 1c po bid ×3w	Take one capsule by mouth twice daily for 3 weeks.
G 1 tsp po q12h prn cong	Give one teaspoon by mouth every 12 hours as needed for congestion.
AAA ud for itching	Apply to affected area(s) as directed for itching.
I 1–2 gtts od qid	Instill one to two drops into left eye four times daily.
I 1P po q12h	Inhale one puff by mouth every 12 hours.

5. After you double-check the information entered into the computer system and know that the information is complete, you can print the label. The label, like the prescription itself, by law must contain certain information, including:

- The name and address of the pharmacy (some states also require the pharmacy phone number)
- The serial or prescription number (as assigned by the computer program)
- The date the prescription was filled (the expiration date is based on the date the prescription was written)

- The name of the prescriber
- The name of the patient
- The name of the drug (some states require both brand and generic names)
- The quantity of drug being dispensed
- Refill information
- Directions for use, including dose and frequency (directions must *not* contain abbreviations)
- Precautions or warnings

6. In many cases, the pharmacy computer will not print a label until the prescription has been charged to the correct party. If the patient has insurance, then the insurance provider has to be billed for this prescription. If the following information has been double-checked, this process will be completed quickly.
    - Patient name and patient or person code
    - Group number and patient ID number
    - Correct number of days' supply
    - NDC number for the medication being dispensed

7. Select, count, and pour the correct medication. Again, the correct medication is verified based on the NDC. A good rule of thumb to ensure that you have the correct drug (other than by NDC) is to read the label three times: once when the drug is selected off the shelf, once when the drug is counted and poured, and once more when the drug is returned to stock. In addition, it is common practice to count twice for accuracy, especially when counting controlled substances.

8. Set up the original prescription or medication order, the stock bottle(s) used, and the finished product for the pharmacist's final approval and verification. For a compounded prescription, the pharmacist will also have to see the recipe sheet you used. Upon successful verification, the pharmacist will approve the medication for dispensing.

9. Store the finished product properly, including patient information sheets, receipts, and notes the pharmacist may need when counseling.

Refilling Prescriptions

A refill is an authorization from the prescriber to fill a prescription exactly as written in addition to the first time it is presented at the pharmacy. A refill allows the patient to receive the medication additional times without the prescriber having to write a new prescription. The expiration date for refills is the same as for the original prescription, and the prescription cannot be dispensed after that date even if the patient has refills remaining.

If the patient has prescription insurance, most plans will pay for a refill only if the patient has used at least 75% of the prescription. The 75% rule is based on the number of days' supply that the technician entered into the computer. Therefore, it is imperative that the days' supply is calculated and entered correctly, or the patient's insurance may not pay for a refill. For example, if the patient receives a 30-day supply of medication on the first day of the month, she must wait at least until the 23rd day of the month before requesting a refill. If she requests a refill earlier, the insurance company will probably reject the claim.

Transferring Prescriptions

The laws governing the transfer of prescriptions between pharmacies differ in various states and depend on the class of drug involved. In most states, it is the pharmacist's responsibility to transfer prescriptions. However, technicians must understand and be familiar with the laws in the state where they practice. Your supervising pharmacist is a great resource to help guide you in transferring prescriptions to or from the pharmacy.

Where it is permitted, a prescription may be transferred for one fill or for the entire prescription. It is important to document the transfer. Both the transferring pharmacy and the receiving pharmacy must keep specific documentation. Check with your state board of pharmacy for specific requirements regarding the transfer of prescriptions in your state.

Once the pharmacy's records show that the prescription was transferred and the prescription has already be filled or refilled, it must be returned to stock. Likewise, any insurance billing claim must be reversed, because two pharmacies cannot charge an insurance company for the same prescription. In such a case, the claim would be rejected.

Compounding Nonsterile Medications

Compounding has always been a basic part of pharmacy practice, even though it has changed a great deal through the years. In the early twentieth century, most prescriptions were compounded in the pharmacy. However, safety and consistency issues arose. For example, without set standards, a prescription for a 500-mg/5-mL suspension may be compounded at 500 mg/5 mL at one pharmacy and at 600 mg/5 ml at another. The number of compounded prescriptions steadily decreased over the decades with the increased availability and mass production of medications.

Today, manufacturers are required by the FDA to follow Good Manufacturing Practices (GMP). GMPs ensure that a 500-mg/-5mL suspension actually contains 500 mg/5 mL. Currently, most pharmacies compound a prescription only if the medication is not available from a manufacturer. When a prescription is compounded for a specific prescription or patient, it is called *extemporaneous compounding*. When a pharmacy compounds medications in anticipation of receiving a prescription, it is called *batch compounding* or *batching*. Batch compounding adds to the pharmacy's inventory and is not intended for a specific prescription or patient.

The number of custom compounding pharmacies is currently on the rise. Physicians, medical institutions, and patients are realizing more than ever the importance of tailoring an individual's medications to meet his or her specific needs. A majority of the pharmacists who are going back to compounding are doing so for love of the science and interest in their patient's well-being. Pharmacists and technicians must ensure that correct drug, dose, and directions are provided, but compounding can often provide the best outcome for the patient.

The following eight factors should be considered when compounding pharmaceuticals.

1. **Organization and Personnel.** The entire pharmacy, including all personnel involved in the manufacturing process, is responsible for producing not only a safe product, but also one that does what it is intended to do. The pharmacists involved have the authority to approve or reject any product manufactured in their facility. The pharmacy also has the responsibility to train technicians or verify that they have the knowledge and skills to perform the duties required.

2. **Facilities.** Compounding and repackaging work areas should be well lit and clean. These areas should be located away from high-traffic areas, public spaces, or any chemicals that might interfere with compounding activities. Ventilation and temperature control also need to be considered.

3. **Equipment.** Equipment must be kept clean and in proper working condition at all times. Pharmacy technicians are usually assigned the tasks of filling, cleaning, and servicing any automated dispensing or compounding systems in a pharmacy practice.

4. **Control of Components and Drug Product Containers and Closures.** An appropriate supply of finished-product containers (vials, lids, suppository molds) and actual drug or drug-component containers (sterile water bottles, simple syrup containers) must be available, and stored in a clean, dust-free environment.

5. **Production and Process Controls.** It is important for good quality control that the medication be made to specific standards and in the same specific way and

proportion each and every time it is manufactured. Recipes may be stored in computers, in notebooks, on cards, and so on. The recipe source should include all ingredients (active and inactive) as well as information on the manner in which the ingredients are combined to ensure strength and purity.

6. **Packaging and Labeling Controls.** It is a good manufacturing practice to monitor package labels constantly to ensure that they contain all the required information and that the information is in the right form. Finished packaging should also be inspected for any defects, such as leaks, cracks, or defective seals. This control process should be addressed in detail in your pharmacy's policies and procedures manual.

7. **Holding and Distribution.** The pharmacy is most likely compounding and manufacturing more than one medication order at a time. Therefore, the finished products must be stored or "quarantined" in such a manner that the medication will not be used until after final verification by the pharmacist. Temperature, humidity, and light must all be considered in medication storage.

8. **Records and Reports.** All compounding processes must be documented and retained, according to state pharmacy law, because there may come a time when a product or even a product container has been recalled and needs to be tracked. Information that needs to be recorded and stored may include:

   • Production dates
   • All components used, including manufacturers, lot numbers, and expiration dates
   • Facility lot number
   • Facility expiration date
   • Identification of equipment used
   • Weights and measures of the components used
   • All in-process quality controls
   • Statement of actual yield
   • Complete labeling control records, including samples of the labels
   • Description of drug product containers and closures
   • Identification of the person(s) performing each step of the process, including final verification

Nonsterile Compounding Equipment

It is a primary duty of a pharmacy technician to maintain all pharmacy equipment. This is especially important in compounding pharmacies, All equipment must remain clean, adjusted, and ready for use at all times. The pharmacist cannot wait while a piece of equipment is located, calibrated, or sanitized. Compounding technicians often use this equipment themselves and must understand its uses and maintenance requirements.

Balances

A Class A (or Class III) prescription balance has two pans and is used for weighing small amounts of drug substances (120 g or less).

The smallest readable amount that can be weighed is 10 mg. This is called the balance's *readability*. The capacity range (CR) for a Class A balance is 60 or 120 g, depending on the balance. The balance's variance or sensitivity requirement (SR) is 6 mg. This is the amount of substance it takes to move the pointer one division mark.

A digital balance is a one-pan balance; the drug is measured inside the wind cover. This type of balance is quickly replacing the prescription balance because is more accurate and easier to use.

Weights

A Class A prescription balance is used with a set of weights. Weights should be stored in their original boxes with clearly marked compartments. Forceps, preferably plastic-tipped, should always be used when handling the weights, because oil from a person's hand can affect the accuracy of the weights. When the scale is in use, the area on which it is placed should be clean, dry, level, and away from air ducts and fans to minimize air movement. When the weights are not in use, they should be properly covered and stored.

Graduated Cylinders

A cylindrical graduated cylinder is designed to have a narrow diameter that is the same from the top to the base. This type of "graduate" can be made out of glass or plastic and is the most commonly used liquid-measuring device in a pharmacy. Selecting the proper graduate depends on the quantity of substance to be measured: The technician should select a cylinder that is only slightly larger than the quantity to be measured. The substance to be measured should never constitute less than 5% of the graduate's capacity.

Compounding Slabs and Ointment Paper

Compounding or ointment slabs are made of ground glass that is approximately ½ to 1 inch thick. They have nonabsorbent surfaces and are used to mix solid and semisolid substances. Most slabs are approximately 12 inches × 12 inches.

Parchment or ointment paper can be used instead of a compounding slab. The advantage to using parchment paper is that there is no clean-up: The paper is discarded after use. A disadvantage is the paper can absorb water when creams are being mixed.

Weigh Papers and Boats

Weigh papers are small, flexible papers that are used to measure and transport powders and semisolid substances. One side is coated with wax to prevent absorption and help to facilitate complete removal of the substance from the paper.

Weigh boats are rigid plastic containers that are used to measure and transport powders and semisolid substances. Most weigh boats have raised edges that make it difficult to completely remove some substances, especially semisolid substances.

Therefore, when measuring semisolid substances, such as ointments, creams, and pastes, it is best to use weigh paper rather than weigh boats. Both weigh papers and wiegh boats are available in a variety of sizes.

Spatulas

Spatulas, available in stainless steel and hard rubber, are used to:

- Count tablets and capsules
- Transfer solid and semisolid ingredients to weighing pans
- Mix liquids and semisolids

The hard rubber spatulas can be porous and can absorb some of the substance. The stainless steel spatulas are less porous but may be corroded by substances such as iodine.

Mortars and Pestles

The most common and recognizable type of pharmacy compounding equipment is the mortar and pestle, which are used to grind, crush, pulverize, and mix pharmaceutical ingredients. The mortar is the cup-shaped vessel in which the materials are ground or crushed, and the pestle is the grinder or pounder. Mortars and pestles are available in glass, wedgewood, and porcelain or ceramic. Glass is preferred for mixing liquids and semisoft dosage forms and are nonporous and nonstaining. Wedgwood has a course surface and arise best for particle reduction. However, it is very porous and stains easily. Wedgwood pestles have wood handles. Porcelain or ceramic have glazed surfaces are considered the standard for pharmacy compounding and particle reduction. The mortar and pestle should always be made of the same material, no matter which type is used.

Compounding Sterile Products

One of the most intricate and demanding tasks a technician can perform is the preparation of intravenous admixtures. Because IVs go directly into a patient's vein, there is no room for error and they must be sterile and prepared under strict United States Pharmacopeia Chapter 797 (USP 797) guidelines. These guidelines are designed to prevent harm or death from contamination, differences in component strengths, contaminants, and inappropriate quality of ingredients for compounded sterile products. USP 797 includes guidelines on the following topics.

- **Compounding Personnel Responsibilities.** This section discusses the responsibilities to ensure that sterile products are compounded, labeled, stored, and dispensed properly.
- **Microbial Contamination Risk Factors.** Based on their potential for contamination, this section categorizes compounded products into low-, medium-, or high-risk-level compounded sterile products and discusses each risk level in detail.
- **Personnel Training and Evaluation in Aseptic Manipulation Skills.** This section provides specific guidelines that personnel should follow to produce a sterile final product.
- **Immediate Use Compounded Sterile Products.** This section details how to handle compounded products that are intended to be used immediately or in emergency situations.
- **Single-Dose and Multiple-Dose Containers.** This section defines the differences between a single- and a multiple-dose container, including expiration dates and time frames.
- **Hazardous Drugs, Radiopharmaceuticals and Allergen Extracts as Compounded Sterile Products.** This section details how, these special types of compounded sterile products should be handled.
- **Verification of Compounding Accuracy of the Sterility of Compounded Sterile Products.** This section discusses in detail the monitoring, testing, and documentation needed to ensure a sterile product.
- **Elements of Quality Control.** This section discusses how specific training and evaluations programs must be developed for all personnel who compound sterile product.
- **Release Checks and Tests.** This section details what types of testing and checks must be performed before a compounded sterile product is dispensed or administered to a patient.
- **Storage and Beyond-Use Dating.** This section details the requirements for storage and expiration dating of compounded sterile products.
- **Maintaining Sterility, Purity, and Stability.** This section discusses how personnel and facilities can maintain sterility, purity, and stability of compounded sterile products during packaging, handling, transportation, use, and storage.
- **Patient or Caregiver Training.** This section details how patients and caregivers should be trained to administer their own compounded sterile products.
- **Patient Monitoring and Adverse Events Reporting.** This section discusses how to monitor and report adverse drug reactions (ADRs).
- **Quality Assurance Program.** This section discusses the characteristics of a compounded sterile product quality-assurance plan.

Admixtures can be compounded in flexible plastic bags, plastic containers, and even glass bottles. The following critical points should be followed when preparing an intravenous admixture to ensure a sterile, effective, and safe sterile product:

- Properly clean and disinfect the compounding areas first with sterile water and low-shedding wipes followed by 70% isopropyl alcohol. The laminar airflow hood should be cleaned at the beginning of each shift. Areas that have direct contact to critical sites such as laminar airflow hoods must be cleaned more frequently than the walls and ceilings of the compounding room.

- Wash hands properly and often. Proper washing of the hands and arms is the technician's best defense against contamination.

- All outer garments (hats, scarves, jackets, etc.) and all hand, wrist, and other visible jewelry, as well as makeup, must be removed before washing hand and donning protective apparel. Artificial or long fingernails should be avoided. Fingernails should be trimmed short.

- Don the appropriate protective apparel in the following order:
  - Shoe covers
  - Head cover and facial hair cover
  - Face mask/eye shield
  - Nonshedding gown
  - Sterile gloves, powder-free

- Before donning the nonshedding gown, the technician must vigorously wash hands and forearms for at least 30 seconds with soap and water.

- After hand washing, don the nonshedding gown and sterile gloves. Clean hands again with a waterless alcohol-based hand scrub. Clean hands throughout the compounding process. Be sure to let gloves dry before beginning manipulations.

- Carefully inspect all ingredients and their containers. Look for cracks, leaks, expiration dates, cloudiness, particulates, and any signs of imperfection.

Sterile Compounding Equipment
Laminar Airflow Hood

The laminar airflow hood (LAH) filters room air twice and keeps the filtered air flowing out toward the operator to prevent any contaminants in the room from entering the work area inside the hood. The primary filters are very similar to regular furnace filters and must be changed or cleaned on a regular basis. The secondary filters in a laminar airflow hood are high-efficiency particulate air (HEPA) filters that remove 99.97% of all particulates that are 0.3 micrometers or larger. Because most airborne contaminants are 0.5 micrometers or larger, the dual filters provide a safe compounding field of 6 inches or more inside the LAH outer edge.

Laminar airflow hoods produce either a horizontal air flow toward the preparer from the back to the front of the hood, or a vertical airflow from the top down to the work surface. Vertical hoods or biological safety cabinets (BSCs) can be used to prepare chemotherapy or hazardous products.

While the hood is in use, nothing should come between the sterile object and the filter (the critical area). In all hoods, objects should be kept 6 inches away from the back and sides of the hood. This allows air to flow freely around the sterile objects. In a vertical airflow system, nothing must be above the object because the airflow is from the top.

If a laminar airflow hood is turned off, it should be turned on for at least 30 minutes before beginning aseptic procedures, including hood cleaning. Pharmacy personnel should change the LAH intake filters every month. In addition, hoods must be inspected and certified by an independent contractor to ensure that they are in proper working order. Hoods must be certified every 6 months, whenever the hood is moved, or whenever it is suspected that they are not working properly.

Needles

Needles are used to transfer liquid medications from one container to another. The needle's *hub* is what attaches the needle to the syringe, and the *shaft* is the long metal part. Needles are measured by gauge and length. *Gauge* is the diameter of the hole or the bore of the needle. The higher the number, the smaller is the gauge. Needles range in size from 13G to 31G with a length of 3/8 to 6 inches.

To maintain sterility, no part of the needle should be touched. The overwrap or protective cover should not be removed until the needle is to be used.

When medication is being drawn from an ampoule, filter needles must be used to protect the patient from any glass fragment that might have fallen into the drug while opening the ampoule. Filter needles have a 5-micrometer filter in the hub.

Syringes

A *syringe* is a device used to inject a sterile solution into an IV bag or directly into the body. The main parts of a syringe are

- The barrel, which holds the medication and is calibrated.
- The plunger, which is used to push fluid in and out of the barrel.
- The tip, which is used to attach the needle to the syringe.

Tips may be Luer-Loc (the needle screws and locks onto the syringe) or slip-tip (the needle slips on the tip but does not lock into place).

Syringes range in size from 0.5 to 60 mL. Syringes are wrapped individually in protective paper or plastic covers. The sterility of the syringe is guaranteed as long as the wrapper is in place and sealed. The syringe seal should not be broken except inside the appropriate compounding area.

It is the responsibility of the technician to choose the correct syringe for the sterile product to be prepared. If you are preparing a nonhazardous medication, choose the syringe closest to the volume being measured. If you are preparing a hazardous medication, use only a Luer-Loc syringe in which the measured volume does not exceed 75% of the capacity of the syringe. For example, to measure 7 mL, you could use a 10-mL syringe, because 7 mL is less than 75% of 10 mL. However, if you need to measure out 8 mL, you will need to use a 20-mL syringe, because 8 mL is more than 75% of 10 mL.

A Patient with a Question but a Busy Pharmacist: Dispensing Information

A dedicated pharmacy technician makes every effort to assist the patient as well as the pharmacist. The technician must have a clear and correct view of what is and what is not appropriate information to dispense. A good rule of thumb is the *single-answer rule:* A question with a single factual answer, such as a drug's alternate name, is usually permissible for a technician to answer. Of course, simple answers, such as the shelf location of an OTC medication or any nonmedical information, can be given freely. In the United States, a technician may never dispense information that requires the professional judgment of a pharmacist. Again, a good rule of thumb is to ask yourself whether there is more than one possible answer. If there is, you must refer the patient to a pharmacist.

It is also important for the technician to know where to find certain pharmaceutical information. The ability to utilize resources not only helps the technician in preparing prescriptions, it is also useful to the pharmacist, who depends on a competent technician to locate certain information for reference before counseling.

The following table lists resources that are commonly found in pharmacies and are available to technicians.

INFORMATION SOURCE	
AHFS (American Hospital Formulary Service) *Drug Information*	Accepted as the authority for drug information questions. Groups monographs by therapeutic use.
American Drug Index	Most exhaustive list of drugs, including drug names, phonetic pronunciations, indications, composition and strengths, dosage forms available, and common abbreviations.
Drug Facts and Comparisons (DFC)	A preferred reference for comprehensive and timely drug information on both prescription and OTC products. Drugs are divided into therapeutic groups, and similar drugs are grouped together in easy-to-use comparative tables. Available in loose-leaf form (with monthly updates), bound yearly editions, and online/CD-ROM (with updates).
FDA *Approved Drug Products with Therapeutic Equivalence Evaluations* (The Orange Book)	Provides information on generic equivalence of drugs. Drugs coded "A" are considered equivalent, drugs coded "B" are not equivalent.
Handbook on Injectable Drugs	Monographs on parenteral (IV) drugs that include concentration, stability, dosage, and compatibility information.
Newsletters	Published rapidly and frequently, these provide a useful source of current information.
Package inserts	Most readily available drug information source for the technician. Required to be included by manufacturers in all drug packages. Package inserts must include the following categories of information: Description; Clinical Pharmacology; Indications and Usage; Contraindications; Warnings and Precautions; Adverse Reactions; Drug Abuse and Dependence; Overdosage; Dosage and Administration; How Supplied; and Date of Revision.
Pharmacy Law Digest of Facts and Comparisons	Provides a general overview of the legal system as it affects pharmacy practice.
Physicians' Desk Reference (PDR)	Annual publication with reprints of package inserts. Contains five color-coded sections: an alphabetical brand-name drug index, a drug classification index by company, a generic and chemical name index, a product identification section, and a product info section of monographs.
Professional practice journals	Official publications of pharmacy organizations, which may reflect the political and policy views of the organization: *Today's Technician* (NPTA), *America's Pharmacist* (NCPA), *American Journal of Health-System Pharmacy* (ASHP), *Journal of the American Pharmacists Association* (APhA).
Red Book: Pharmacy's Fundamental Reference	Product information on legend, OTC, and reimbursable medical supplies, including the latest pricing, average wholesale price (AWP) and suggested retail. Includes National Drug Code (NDC) numbers for all FDA-approved drugs.
The Merck Index	Encyclopedic source of chemicals, drugs, and biological, containing monographs referenced by trade, code, chemical, investigational, and abbreviated drug names.
The Merck Manual	The most widely used medical reference, it includes information on diagnosis and treatment.
The Science and Practice of Pharmacy (Remington's)	The most comprehensive text in the pharmaceutical sciences, covering all aspects of pharmacy including evolution of pharmacy, ethics, pharmaceutics, pharmaceutical testing and manufacturing, pharmacodynamics, and pharmacy practice. Revised every five years.
Trade journals	Published for pharmacy but not by the profession: *American Druggist, Pharmacy Times, Drug Topics,* and *US Pharmacists.*
United States Pharmacopeia Drug Information (USP DI)	Comprehensive and clinically relevant information on current drugs. Divided into three volumes: Vol. I, *Drug Information for the Health Care Professional;* Vol. II, *Advice for the Patient;* Vol. III, *Approved Drug Products and Legal Requirements.*

Governmental, professional, and pharmacy organizations are also good sources of information for the pharmacy technician. The following table lists organizations the pharmacy technician should be familiar with.

ORGANIZATION NAME AND ACRONYM	PURPOSE/FUNCTION
American Association of Colleges of Pharmacy (AACP)	Represents all 88 pharmacy schools and represents the interests of pharmaceutical education & educators. Publishes the *American Journal of Pharmaceutical Education.*
American Association of Pharmacy Technicians (AAPT)	National organization that represents technicians. Established/developed the Pharmacy Technician Code of Ethics.
Accreditation Council for Pharmacy Education (ACPE)	The national agency for the accreditation of professional degree programs in pharmacy and providers of continuing pharmacy education.
American Pharmacists Association (APhA)	Largest national pharmacy organization representing the interests of pharmacists.
American Society of Health-System Pharmacists (ASHP)	National organization that represents pharmacists and technicians in institutional settings (hospitals, HMOs, long-term care, home care). Accrediting agency for pharmacy residency and pharmacy technician programs.
Centers for Disease Control and Prevention (CDC)	Part of the U.S. Department of Health and Human Services, the CDC collaborates to create the expertise, information, and tools that people and communities need to protect their health, through health promotion, prevention of disease, injury, and disability, and preparedness for new health threats. The CDC monitors health, detects and investigates health problems, conducts research to enhance prevention, develops and advocates sound public health policies, implements prevention strategies, and promotes healthy behaviors.
Drug Enforcement Administration (DEA)	Federal agency that enforces controlled-substances laws and regulations by bringing any organization or person involved in the growing, manufacture, or distribution of controlled substances appearing in or destined for illicit traffic into the U.S. criminal and civil court system.
Food and Drug Administration (FDA)	Federal agency responsible for ensuring that foods are safe, wholesome, and sanitary; human and veterinary drugs, biological products, and medical devices are safe and effective; cosmetics are safe; and electronic products that emit radiation are safe. The FDA also ensures that these products are represented to the public honestly, accurately, and informatively.
Occupational Safety and Health Administration (OSHA)	Part of the U.S. Department of Labor, its mission is to prevent work-related injuries, illnesses, and deaths. OSHA establishes and enforces workplace safety standards.
National Pharmacy Technician Association (NPTA)	World's largest professional organization established specifically for pharmacy technicians. The association is dedicated to advancing the value of pharmacy technicians and the vital roles they play in pharmaceutical care.
Pharmacy Technician Educators Council (PTEC)	National Organization of educators who prepare people to become pharmacy technicians.
The Joint Commission (formerly JCAHO)	Establishes standards intended to improve the quality and safety of patient care. The Joint Commission sets standards and accredits health care providers and evaluates performance through on-site inspections.
United States Pharmacopeia (USP)	Nonprofit organization that sets standards for the identity, strength, quality, purity, packaging, and labeling of drug products. Publishes the USP 797 guidelines for sterile compounding.

Adjudication

Another valuable service to both patients and pharmacists that a technician provides is adjudication. *Adjudication* is the processing of an insurance claim or bill. In retail, before a drug is delivered to a patient, the billing must be completed or the patient must pay for the prescription. Computer adjudication programs perform this process.

For insurance billing, proper prescription screening is very important. In order to bill an insurance company, the technician must have all the pertinent information, including the patient's full name, date of birth, and account number. Hospital billing is similar, but there are some differences. First, in retail the pharmacy transmits the charges for the entire prescription to the patient or the patient's insurance. In a hospital, the pharmacy inputs daily patient charges for the drugs used, and this information is then transmitted to the hospital billing department. It is the billing department that actually sends the bills to the patient or the insurance company, not the pharmacy. It is easy to understand that entering all pertinent profile information and prescription information correctly is a critical responsibility of the technician. If this process is not handled properly, billing errors, profile duplications, and insurance denials may occur, and the pharmacy may not receive payment for medications that have been dispensed.

Collecting from a Third Party

Third-party billing is a system in which a third party, usually an insurance carrier, pays the pharmacy for services rendered to a patient. The insurance carrier is paid a monthly premium by the patient or the patient's employer. The pharmacy bills the carrier at the time of sale, and the patient pays any deductible or co-payment at the same time.

Co-Payments

Co-payments or "co-pays" are fees paid directly to the pharmacy by the patient when a medication is dispensed. Co-pays are set flat fees that the patient pays for each prescription filled, regardless of the cost of the medication. Patients may be responsible for different co-pays depending on whether the prescription is for a generic or a brand-name drug. For example, a patient may pay $5.00 for generic and $15.00 for brand-name drugs. A *tiered co-pay* increases as it moves from generic to preferred brand to nonpreferred brand (a patient pays, say, $10.00 for generic, $20.00 for a preferred brand, and $40.00 for a nonpreferred brand).

Co-Insurance

Co-insurance is a percentage of the cost that a patient pays for a specific drug or service. Co-insurance rates are preset by the insurance company but, unlike co-pays, the amount the patient pays is based on the price of the drug or service. For example, if a patient has a 10% co-insurance clause in his policy, he will pay $5.00 for a $50.00 generic prescription.

Spend-Downs and Deductibles

Spend-downs and deductibles are also sources of out-of-pocket expense to the patient. Spend-downs or deductibles are preset yearly costs that a patient must pay before the third party pays anything toward the costs of prescriptions.

Insurance Responses and Denials

Insurance billing can be a challenging part of a pharmacy technician's daily duties, but if it is done correctly, it provides a tremendous service to the patient. Most pharmacies have computerized point-of-sale (POS) billing, which means that the insurance company is petitioned and approves payment to the pharmacy at the time of dispensing and before the patient receives the medication.

Of course, the technician must start with the correct patient and patient information. Sometimes there may be glitches, challenges, or denials on the part of the insurance company. A good technician learns to deal with these in a calm, professional, and determined manner. The following are some common alert messages that a technician may see while processing the insurance billing for a prescription.

- **"Patient Not Eligible."** This might mean that some piece of information in the patient's profile is incorrect. Check spelling of name, date of birth, patient code, and whether the correct insurance company is being billed.
- **"Refill Too Soon."** A prescription with refills remaining can usually be refilled when 75% percent of the medication has been used, but not before. This is why the date written and days' supply must be entered accurately. For example, if Mr. Schmidt was given a prescription for 15 tablets and the directions read, "Take 1 tablet each day," and the technician enters 30 as the days' supply, then "refill too soon" will be the insurance company's reply when Mr. Schmidt returns for a refill. A good technician will be able to detect the problem quickly and correct it.
- **"Medication Not Covered."** Insurance companies have formularies of approved drugs, which are constantly changing. A "medication not covered" message means that the drug that is being billed is not covered by the patient's insurance company. The patient can still get the prescription filled, but she must pay for it herself. At this point, the technician should alert the pharmacist.
- **"Prior Authorization Required."** Many insurance companies require that a review be conducted before medications are dispensed or prescribed. If a patient presents a prescription to the pharmacy without review by the insurance company, the pharmacy technician will receive the message "prior authorization required."

SUMMARY

By definition, pharmacy technicians are employed to assist pharmacists in providing safe and efficient pharmaceutical care, which makes it is easy to understand why this area is so heavily weighted on the certification exam.

Remember, 66% of the exam relates to this topic—in other words, roughly 60 of the 90 test questions will be based on the material in this chapter.

CHAPTER REVIEW QUESTIONS

1. A primary duty of a pharmacy technician is patient counseling.
   a. true
   b. false

2. The day-to-day management of quality in the pharmacy is known as:
   a. quality assurance
   b. quality control
   c. quality improvement
   d. quality management

3. What part of a prescription identifies how often the drug should be taken or administered?
   a. dosage form
   b. route of administration
   c. schedule
   d. patient dose
   e. drug strength

4. What part of a prescription identifies the potency of the drug to be dispensed?
   a. dosage form
   b. route of administration
   c. schedule
   d. patient dose
   e. drug strength

5. Could DEA# BM1467821 be correct for a prescription written by Dr. Mary Jones?
   a. yes
   b. no

6. Patient allergies will most likely be found in what part of the patient profile?
   a. demographic info
   b. prescription history
   c. prescription preferences
   d. medical history
   e. insurance information

7. Technicians are generally allowed to bypass clinical warnings when entering prescriptions.
   a. true
   b. false

8. The bolded section of NDC 0001-00-01 identifies:
   a. the manufacturer
   b. the package size
   c. the dosage form and strength
   d. the distributor
   e. both a and d

9. The abbreviation BID stands for:
   a. once daily
   b. twice daily
   c. three times daily
   d. four times daily

10. Which of the following information is *not* required to be on a written prescription?
    a. patient name
    b. date written
    c. doctor's signature
    d. diagnosis
    e. drug name

11. Of the following information, which is required to be on a prescription label?
    a. name of pharmacy
    b. name of patient
    c. quantity of drug dispensed
    d. name of prescriber
    e. all the above

12. The best way to ensure that you have chosen the correct drug to fill a prescription is by:
    a. choosing the drug by the color of the label
    b. choosing the drug by the generic name
    c. choosing the drug based on the NDC
    d. choosing the drug based on the shape of the tablet

13. At a minimum, a pharmacy technician should read the drug label ____ times to help avoid filling errors.
    a. 1
    b. 2
    c. 3
    d. 4

14. Which organization requires pharmacies to follow GMPs when compounding nonsterile products?
    a. FDA
    b. ASHP
    c. USP
    d. DEA

15. The bolded section of NDC **0001**–00-01 is called the _____ code:
    a. package code
    b. product code
    c. labeler code
    d. none of the above

16. Which organization has established national guidelines for compounding sterile products?
    a. FDA
    b. ASHP
    c. USP
    d. DEA

17. Which type of mortar and pestle is preferred for mixing liquids?
    a. porcelain
    b. ceramic
    c. wedgewood
    d. glass

18. USP 797 has guidelines in place to ensure the correct handling of compounded sterile products used in emergency situations.
    a. true
    b. false

19. USP 797 requires that compounding areas be first cleaned with:
    a. soap and water
    b. sterile water
    c. 70% isopropyl alcohol
    d. none of the above

20. According to USP 797, the technician should don which of the following last?
    a. hair cover
    b. face mask
    c. sterile gloves
    d. gown
    e. shoe covers

3

Maintaining Medication/Inventory Control

After completing this chapter, you should be able to:

- Define *inventory* and understand the differences between inventory management and inventory control.
- Explain the role of the formulary in maintaining drug inventories.
- Describe and compare the various inventory management systems used in pharmacy settings.
- List the steps for returning outdated or misordered drugs.
- Describe the drug recall process.
- Compare the processes used in ordering and inventory of controlled substances to those for ordering other drugs.
- Describe the storage and disposal requirements for investigational and compounded medications.
- Describe and explain the Controlled Substances Act (CSA), and list and describe the five drug classes.
- Describe the two primary types of inventory management systems: manual and point-of-sale (POS).
- Explain how to assist with special ordering and receiving procedures.
- Explain medication storage and distribution.
- Describe safe handling of cytotoxic and hazardous materials.
- Discuss special concerns regarding controlled substances and investigational drugs.
- Explain bulk compounding and repackaging of pharmaceuticals.

Introduction

In the practice of pharmacy, inventory control is one of the most important responsibilities of pharmacy technicians, and the quality and quantity of products can mean the difference between life and death for patients. One can easily see, then, why monitoring the purchase, storage, and quantities of drugs and supplies is part of protecting the health of the public, just as much as dispensing the correct drug to the right patient.

To meet patient needs, medications have to be on hand and in proper condition. On the other hand, certain medications can be very expensive and costly to store. Medications also have expiration dates beyond which they cannot be used or dispensed. So inventory control is a sort of balancing act that requires great attention to detail.

First, the drugs and/or ingredients must be purchased and shipped to the pharmacy. To get started, the pharmacy must have a Drug Enforcement Administration (DEA) number assigned to it. Second, a source or supplier must be selected. Technically, a pharmacy can purchase directly from each manufacturer, but that would be time-consuming and paperwork-prohibitive.

For this reason, pharmacies usually contract with a primary wholesaler to obtain many different manufacturers' products from one supplier. When a pharmacy agrees to purchase 80–90% of all its pharmaceuticals from a single wholesaler, that wholesaler is termed a *prime vendor*. The wholesaler acts as an intermediary in procuring pharmaceuticals and other supplies for the pharmacy at special prices. This agreement still allows the pharmacy to make special purchases from other vendors when necessary. The wholesaler gets shipments directly from numerous manufacturers and can provide their products to the pharmacy all charged on one convenient invoice.

Although the pharmacist in charge (PIC) is ultimately responsible for overseeing inventory management and control, day-to-day management tasks such as ordering, receiving, and control process are generally handled by a pharmacy technician.

Inventory Control
The Formulary System

There are so many drugs on the market today, with so many uses, that it would be counterproductive to stock all of them in any one pharmacy setting. So how does a pharmacy know what to stock? The answer is a *formulary,* a list of all the drugs, medications, and devices approved for dispensing from your pharmacy.

In hospitals, a pharmacy and therapeutics (P&T) committee determines the formulary. The committee meets several times each year and discusses which medications are appropriate for treatment of various disease states and conditions. It is the committee's responsibility to keep up with the ever-changing information on the newest and most effective drugs for various conditions and disease states, taking note of research and changing conditions in the health care industry. The committee arrives at an approved list of medications, weighted with the cost of each medication, to be used at that particular facility.

In most retail settings, a buyer or head pharmacist usually makes that decision for all the pharmacies under his or her authority. However, in an independent retail setting, it is the owner's responsibility.

Regardless of who makes the decision, six key components lead to the final decision:

- Drug availability
- Dosage form
- Strength or concentration
- Accepted therapeutic uses
- Correct dosages
- Federal, state, or local policy affecting the use of a medication (such as a restricted antibiotic)

Inventory Management Systems

Pharmacy technicians maintain all aspects of a pharmacy's inventory. Using the formulary as a guide, the technician must ensure that adequate stock of all medication and medical devices will be available between deliveries. The technician must also monitor the expiration dates of current stock levels and see to the proper storage of all drugs and medication components in the pharmacy. This will ensure that all drugs in the pharmacy are safe and effective. The system used by the technician to accomplish all this is called an inventory control or management system.

Two main types of inventory management systems are used by pharmacies: manual and computerized or point-of-sale (POS) systems.

Smaller pharmacies may use a manual inventory management system, whereas larger retail pharmacies and hospital pharmacies use computerized systems that automatically record all inventory transactions.

A computerized or point-of-sale inventory system works much like a balance sheet, as each drug or medication component on the shelves is tracked from the time it is ordered to the time it is dispensed. As medications are dispensed, the computer subtracts those drugs from the inventory; when new drugs are received, it adds those medications to the inventory. POS systems automatically create medication orders based on the pharmacy's use of drugs.

A pharmacy technician who uses a POS system does not need to do a physical inventory before each order but must review the computer-generated order for accuracy before it is transmitted. If demand for a medication increases, the technician can adjust the order point accordingly. The *minimum order point* is the amount of a product left on the shelf that will automatically trigger a reorder. The *maximum order level* indicates the maximum quantity that should be on the shelf at any one time. Order levels are determined based on drug usage, and these levels reflect the smallest and largest quantities of a drug or medication component to be kept on the shelves. Once the minimum quantity is reached (or approached), the computer automatically adds the item to the order list. A pharmacy's inventory costs money to maintain. To keep costs and waste down, inventory must be kept at a level that will ensure that the pharmacy will not run out of a drug before the next order arrives, but not so high that it means unnecessary costs to the pharmacy. For example, if Mary knows that her pharmacy dispenses about 100 units of warfarin each week, she may set the order point at 25 units. The computer will automatically reorder warfarin when the inventory reaches or falls below 25 units. The minimum and maximum inventory levels will increase or decrease as usage of the medication increases or decreases.

A manual system requires all inventory activities to be done by hand. A physical inventory is taken at regular intervals, and a decision is made as to what needs to be ordered. Often, a "want book" is used to determine what drugs need to be ordered. A "want book" is a place where technicians and pharmacists can write down which drugs are low or out of stock when they dispense them. With a manual system, the inventory technician needs to be very familiar with the movement of each drug and decide how much of that drug is enough to last until the arrival of the next delivery. Manual ordering systems are generally used in smaller pharmacies, where the volume of inventory is lower.

It is even more important that the inventory technician is diligent in maintaining correct inventory levels of all drugs, medications, equipment, and components. A manual ordering system works on the same basic principles as an automated ordering system, but without the advantage of the computer. A technician using a manual ordering system must follow the pharmacy's formulary, set order levels, and manually create an inventory order, which is then usually transmitted over the phone. Stock rotation and order-level adjustments are also completed on a regular basis using both automated and manual systems.

Purchasing

Whether the order was compiled electronically or manually, the technician must arrange for the purchase. Several options are available to all pharmacies. A pharmacy may purchase drugs directly from the manufacturer, from a wholesaler, or from other vendors. Pharmacy management, not technicians, decides where the drug will be ordered from. To place a drug order, the technician must create a purchase order (PO). An order cannot be processed without a purchase order that contains at least the following information:

- Name of drug
- Dosage form
- Package size
- Concentration/strength
- Quantity of each package
- Drug identification or NDC number

The PO will also contain the pharmacy name, address, phone number, and customer ID number. Electronic ordering will automatically transmit the pertinent pharmacy information along with the actual order. In many cases, manual ordering is done on preprinted forms, with several copies for each order.

If the pharmacy is ordering from a manufacturer, the pharmacy fills out a purchase order and sends it directly to the manufacturer. Once the order is received, the manufacturer fills the order and sends it to the pharmacy. This is an example of a *direct purchase*.

In purchasing, there is strength in numbers, and sometimes pharmacies band together and make a commitment to a manufacturer to purchase large quantities of drugs, medications, and supplies over a period of a year or more. The manufacturer, in turn, reduces the cost of drugs to pharmacies in this group. This is an example of buying drugs through a *purchasing group*.

Most retail pharmacies purchase inventory through wholesale purchasing. The wholesaler purchases drugs, medications, and supplies from many different manufacturers and warehouses them at one location. Most pharmacies are able to purchase 85–95% of their inventories from this single source. They usually cannot purchase 100% of their inventories from any one supplier because of special-order items or items that may be needed but not supplied by that wholesaler.

Receiving an Order

Once the order has been placed, the pharmacy awaits its arrival. Most wholesale pharmacy suppliers deliver two or more times per day, and most orders are received within 24 hours of placing the order. This enables pharmacies to have a smaller inventory and still ensure that patients get their medications promptly. Many suppliers deliver on a daily basis, and some even provide for weekend delivery for pharmacies that operate on a 24/7 schedule. On the other hand, ordering direct from the manufacturer takes longer, depending on the ordering relationship between the manufacturer and the pharmacy.

Medications are delivered in medication totes or boxes. Usually included in the delivery of medication are the corresponding packing slips and invoices. Packing slips are used by the wholesaler to pull and pack the drug order. Invoices are used to bill the pharmacy for the medications that have been ordered and delivered.

Controlled substances are listed on a separate invoice and packed in a separate container from other drugs, and delivery must be verified by a pharmacist. Chemotherapy and refrigerated/frozen medications also arrive in a separate container.

Along with the invoices, stickers are often included with the order. These stickers facilitate easier reordering, especially under a manual system, because important information is printed on each specific item's sticker. As items are checked line by line against the invoice, price stickers are affixed to the product itself. When affixing stickers, it is important not to cover any information such as the drug name, strength, and lot number or expiration date. Most inventory stickers include the following information:

- Wholesaler's item number
- Date of receipt
- Net cost
- Average wholesale price (AWP)
- Invoice number

Careful checking of each item is imperative to make sure that only those items received are added to the pharmacy's inventory. Receiving an item into the inventory that was not actually shipped is one of the most common errors under a point-of-sale system. The result is a shortage of medication that may or may not be realized until that particular medication is needed for a patient.

Receiving and stocking inventory are two of the most important responsibilities of the entire pharmacy inventory operation. Mistakes made during this process can easily jeopardize the health of patients and produce costly consequences.

It is important that all stock be completely checked against the invoice when it is delivered. The following is a step-by-step approach that should be followed when receiving inventory.

1. Make sure that the name and address on the boxes is correct. Drug deliveries often end up at the wrong location, especially with chain store deliveries.
2. Make sure that the shipping manifest of the carrier matches the actual number of boxes delivered. All boxes should be accounted for. For example, if the invoice indicates five boxes, your first task is to verify that there are five boxes. Quickly check the boxes for any signs of leakage or damage and then sign for delivery of the order.
3. Retrieve the manufacturer or warehouse invoice and/or packing slip; if any box or container is marked to be refrigerated or kept frozen, immediately place the contents in the refrigerator or freezer to avoid product damage. Special order, chemotherapy, and investigational drugs should be handled according to facility protocol.
4. The following information should be checked against the purchase order or invoice:
   - Name of drug
   - NDC
   - Strength/dosage
   - Dosage form
   - Quantity
   - Expiration date (Checking the expiration date is extremely important: Drugs with short dating should be returned to the supplier for items with longer dating.)
5. Once the order has been confirmed as correct, the new stock is almost ready to be put on the shelves. First, though, the inventory labels must be attached (in most cases, to the bottom of the container). As the technician puts the labeled

medications in the correct storage areas, he or she should rotate stock (put items with shorter expiration dates at the front of the shelf or bin, items with longer expiration dates at the back). Rotating stock this way helps to avoid accumulating expired drugs, which might be dispensed accidentally.

Removing Stock from Inventory

One of the main priorities of inventory control is to make sure that the inventory is in usable condition and safe for patient use. Recalled, expired, and improperly stored drugs must be immediately removed from the pharmacy inventory.

Routine expiration date and/or storage audits must be conducted of the medication inventory stock in both retail and hospital pharmacies, because the pharmacy is responsible for medication control of the entire facility. During these audits the technician checks for drugs that have expired or will soon expire, and for any drugs that may be stored improperly.

In hospitals, these audits are commonly called *nursing station inspections*. The central pharmacy, satellite pharmacies, nursing units, patient care areas, and any other locations where drugs are stored in the facility must be included in these audits.

These routine audits may be done on a monthly or quarterly basis, depending on facility protocol. Written documentation showing the results of these audits should be kept available for review if needed.

Recalls

In compliance with Article 20 of the FDA's Pharmaceutical Good Manufacturing Practices, an alert system must be in place to notify proper authorities in the event of a pharmaceutical recall. The goal of the alert system is to protect the public's health from potential risks caused by using defective or unsafe pharmaceutical products.

A recall is an event in which a firm (a supplier or manufacturer) agrees to remove and correct marketed products that are in violation of applicable laws, may be defective, or may pose a potential risk to the health of the public. There may be many different reasons for recall of a pharmaceutical product. Common reasons for recalls include quality defects, contamination, and counterfeiting.

Recalls are classified according to the relative degree of health hazard of the product that is being recalled. The classifications are divided into three groups: Class I, Class II, and Class III.

- In Class I recalls, the use of or exposure to a particular product is likely to cause serious adverse health consequences or even death. It is the most severe of the three classes.

- In Class II recalls, the use of or exposure to a particular product may cause temporary harm or medically reversible adverse health consequences, or the likelihood of serious adverse health consequences is very remote.

- In Class III recalls, the use of or exposure to a particular product is not likely to cause serious adverse health consequences.

In the event of a recall, the FDA forwards a recall notice containing pertinent information the pharmacy needs to take appropriate action. Recall notices include the following information:

- Recall classification
- Recall number
- Product name
- Dosage form and strength of the medication
- Packaging information (size)
- Batch or lot control numbers affected by the recall
- Expiration dates

- Brief description or reason for the recall
- Product manufacturer's name and address

Upon receiving such information, the inventory control manager should check the information given in the recall against the inventory in stock. Any recalled products in stock should be promptly removed from the inventory. Appropriate instructions will be included with the recall information as to what actions to take in returning the recalled product(s) to the manufacturer or drug wholesaler.

Medications that are unsafe for patient use, including expired and recalled products, should be segregated from other medications. The storage area for these medications should be labeled as such, so that the chance of using unsafe products is eliminated.

In many cases, the recall process begins with the FDA's MedWatch program. MedWatch is a program under which health care professionals and consumers voluntarily report serious adverse events, product quality problems, product use errors, or therapeutic inequivalence/failures that are suspected or known to be associated with the use of an FDA-regulated drug, biologic, medical device, dietary supplement, or cosmetic. Suspected counterfeit medical products are also reported to the FDA through MedWatch.

Returns

Each wholesaler has its own policies for accepting returned merchandise and drug products for either replacement or credit. First, authorization must be obtained from the supplier for the return, and then that supplier's specific return procedure must be followed.

Expired Drugs

Despite careful ordering and product rotation, a drug will sometimes expire before it can be dispensed. In some cases, these drugs may be returned to the supplier for credit. In other cases, they must simply be destroyed. Authorizations and forms need to be completed before the products can be packaged and shipped. Pharmacies sometimes hire a "returns company," which, for a fee, goes through all the pharmacy shelves and collects expired and unusable drugs, fills out the appropriate paperwork, and packages the drugs for shipment back to the supplier.

Controlled Substances

Under the federal Controlled Substances Act (CSA), all drugs under federal control are placed into one of five schedules or categories. The factors that determine where a drug is ranked for scheduling purposes include medicinal value, harmfulness, and potential for abuse. A pharmacy technician should be aware of the schedules of drugs and their potential for danger or abuse.

Drugs in Schedule I have no medicinal value. Drugs in this class are illicit or "street" drugs such as heroin, cocaine, and LSD.

Schedule II includes a number of drugs that pharmacies dispense on a daily basis. Included in this class are stimulants such as methylphenidate (Concerta, Ritalin) and severe-pain medications such as oxycodone (Percocet, Tylox), morphine sulfate (Avinza, Roxanol), meperidine (Demerol), and fentanyl (Sublimaze). The Schedule II medications are the drugs in a pharmacy that are kept under the highest level of security and regulation. Obtaining them for patient use is more complex than obtaining other drugs.

Medications in Schedule III (e.g., Vicodin, Tylenol #3, testosterone), Schedule IV (e.g., Valium, Xanax, Lunesta), and Schedule V (e.g., cough syrups with codeine) require a different level of control because of their lower risk of danger and abuse potential. These drugs, which include pain medications as well as antianxiety and antidepressant agents, still require high security levels. Although obtaining them may not be as complex as obtaining Schedule II drugs, they are still controlled substances and are regulated more than noncontrolled drugs.

Distribution throughout the facility should be monitored properly so that all controlled substances can be accounted for at all times. Excellent and up-to-date record-keeping is a must in order to maintain an accurate count of all drugs with controlled status.

With manual accounting systems, paper documentation of controlled-drug distribution must be kept on file in the pharmacy. Where drugs are stored in automated dispensing systems, computerized records are available for documentation purposes. With either system, basically the same information is needed for access to controlled substances.

When these drugs are distributed from the pharmacy to a nursing unit or other patient care area, they are logged from inventory onto a "sign-out" sheet. If automated technologies are employed, the logging-out process may be done electronically.

Procedures for controlled-substance distribution may vary slightly from one health system to another, but they all adhere closely to the standard principles and requirements.

Controlled substances in Schedules III, IV, and V can be ordered along with the pharmacy's regular order. They are automatically invoice separately because of their controlled status. These drugs are shipped to the pharmacy in separate containers from all other medications. Although a pharmacy technician may oversee the receiving of all other medications, a licensed pharmacist should verify incoming controlled substances.

Schedule II Drugs

Schedule II drugs (also called C-II drugs) have very specific ordering, receiving, storage, dispensing, inventory, record-keeping, return, waste, and disposal requirements mandated by federal law. Because of their high potential for abuse, the Drug Enforcement Administration (DEA) makes obtaining them more complex than obtaining other medications. The DEA, a division of the U.S. Department of Justice, requires a special form (DEA Form 222) for procurement of C-II medications from a supplier.

Only a pharmacy with a DEA number is allowed to order and dispense Schedule II medications, just as only a prescriber with a DEA number can prescribe them. Even though a purchasing and inventory technician may actually fill out the form, the person with power of attorney must sign it and is the only person who may sign a DEA Form 222. In most instances, it is a pharmacist who has the authority to sign the DEA Form 222. The DEA's Controlled Substance Ordering System (CSOS) allows for electronic orders of controlled substances without requiring a paper form DEA 222.

DEA Form 222 contains ten lines on three copies (the original, which is brown, copy 2, which is green, and copy 3, which is blue). After the form is filled out by the pharmacy, the brown and green copies are sent to the supplier, while the blue copy is kept by the pharmacy for its records. The supplier fills the order, keeps the original brown copy, and sends the green copy to the DEA for drug-tracking purposes. The DEA can track a C-II drug from its manufacturing site to the supplier, to the pharmacy, and to the patient. Each dose must be accounted for at all times and at every stage of the distribution process.

Filling out a DEA Form 222 is a precise undertaking; if a mistake is made, a new form must be completed. There can be no cross-outs or changes of any kind on a DEA Form 222. These important guidelines must be followed:

- Only pen or typewriter may be used.
- Only one drug may be ordered per line.
- The signature on the DEA Form 222 must match that on the DEA license or power-of-attorney form.
- The third copy must be kept for two years and must be kept separate from other records and/or forms.

There can be no changes, erasures, or cross-outs. Incorrect forms must be marked *VOID* and kept with the other DEA Form 222s. When the C-II drugs are delivered, the person receiving the delivery must be 18 years old, and the date received must be written on the pharmacy's copy. Federal law requires all Form 222s to be kept on file for two years. State law may require a longer holding period. Pharmacies are also required to keep separate C-II inventory logs as well as separate storage of C-II prescriptions or dispensing records.

Expired C-II drugs cannot be returned to the manufacturer or wholesaler for credit. Expired C-II drugs must be destroyed, often by a specially licensed company, and recorded on the separate DEA Form 41. DEA Form 41, "Registrants Inventory of Drug Surrendered," is used to inventory and record any C-II drug that must be destroyed. If there is a suspected theft or loss of a controlled substance, DEA Form 160, "The Report of Theft or Loss of Controlled Substances," must be completed. Technicians work closely with a pharmacist when handling any C-II drug and C-II paperwork.

Investigational Drugs

Certain hospitals or institutional pharmacies may handle investigational medications. Only a licensed physician may initiate the request for such a drug. The first step is to obtain permission from the manufacturer. Without this permission, the unapproved product cannot be made available to patients.

These drugs are tracked with a perpetual inventory system that is usually maintained by pharmacy technicians. Instructions are provided that cover the receiving, storage, and return of investigational drugs by the manufacturer or the sponsor of the study.

Investigational drugs that have expired or become unstable should not be thrown away but kept, clearly marked, and handled according to instructions from the manufacturer or sponsor of the study.

Compounded Drugs

Compounded drugs or medications manufactured in a pharmacy usually have strict storage requirements and short expiration dates. Technicians must monitor the production levels, storage, and waste of these materials. The technician must be aware of the employer's policy on the disposal of expired compounded medications and must follow that policy.

Other Inventory Issues

Other medications that have special ordering procedures may require a pharmacy representative to call the manufacturer or wholesaler to provide specific information pertaining to the medication or its use. A few examples are Embrel injection and Thalomid tablets. Sometimes these specially ordered products are not kept in stock at the wholesaler's warehouse, but are *drop-shipped* from the manufacturer, which means that the order is billed or charged by the wholesaler but shipped from a different location, such as from the manufacturer.

Medication availability is also a primary concern of purchasing and inventory technicians. To stay abreast of situations such as drug shortages, the pharmacy buyer should be well aware of all that is going on within the pharmacy inventory and at the wholesaler. Some key terms dealing with medication availability need to be understood.

The inventory technician may find a drug that is "temporarily out of stock." This means that the supplier is out of the medication and expects a shipment from the manufacturer within a short time. If a medication is out of stock, the pharmacy can wait until the drug is received from the wholesaler or, if it is needed immediately, the pharmacy can "borrow" the medication from another pharmacy and "repay" the pharmacy when a shipment is received.

On the other hand, a "manufacturer back order" happens when the wholesaler is out of the product and none is available from the manufacturer. A back order may last a few days, weeks, or even months. A back order might result from a shutdown of manufacturing, a recall, or even a raw material shortage. When an out-of-stock or back order occurs, it is the responsibility of the inventory technician and the pharmacist to decide if an alternate manufacturer or an alternate drug should be ordered.

Medication Storage

Medication storage is a very important part of controlling inventory. It is necessary to provide the correct environment for medications and components until they are needed, so that they maintain their potency and stability. If proper environmental control is not maintained, the medications may not be safe and effective for patient use. Factors that affect the environment include:

- Temperature
- Light
- Humidity
- Ventilation
- Sanitation
- Segregation

In a retail pharmacy, medications are stored primarily on the pharmacy inventory shelves. In a hospital setting, medications may be stored in several different areas throughout the institution or outpatient pharmacy, including:

- Pharmacy shelves (in both central and satellite pharmacies)
- Refrigerators
- Nursing units and automated dispensing systems
- Clinics and treatment rooms
- Emergency, operating, and recovery rooms

No matter where drugs are located in the facility, the responsibility for all medications falls on the shoulders of the pharmacy workers, particularly those who work with inventory management and control. Storage areas must be secure and accessible only to designated and authorized personnel. Whenever possible, records should be kept of who has accessed the medication storage areas. Areas such as automated dispensing systems, after-hours cabinets, and locked cabinets containing controlled substances are prime areas for such access monitoring.

Segregation of pharmacy supplies and medications should be a high priority. External-use products should be stored separately from internal-use products, just as nasal and inhalation products should be kept separate from otic and ophthalmic preparations. This segregation is required by the Joint Commission to help prevent medication errors and improper use of medications.

Some of the main segregated areas of the pharmacy include areas for:

- Oral tablets, capsules, and powders
- Oral liquids, including solutions, elixirs, syrups, and undiluted antibiotic suspensions
- Topicals, including creams, ointments, and patches
- Ophthalmic medications
- Otic medications
- Orally inhaled medications
- Nasal products
- Rectal suppositories and topical rectal preparations
- Vaginal products
- Injectables
- Cytotoxic medications
- Other hazardous chemicals

In general, most pharmacy inventory storage is by drug generic name in the appropriate area of the pharmacy. For example, atenolol tablets are stored in the A section of tablets, capsules, and powders. Also located in that same area, next to the atenolol, will be the trade-name Tenormin tablets if that is also a stock item. However, some pharmacies may store inventory alphabetically by trade name. In such a pharmacy, Tenormin tablets would be stored in the T section, and the atenolol would be stored right next to them. This storage method is quickly fading away, however, because of the vast majority of products now becoming available in generic form. In other pharmacies, the Tenormin might be shelved in the T section and the atenolol in the A section. This method is used only in retail pharmacies.

Storage temperature can greatly affect the stability and potency of a medication. Pharmaceuticals are labeled to show the required temperature range for their proper storage. The most common temperature storage requirements are as follows:

- Room temperature (59–86°F or 15–30°C):

  Most tablets, powders, capsules, and liquids

- Refrigerator (36–46°F or 2–8°C):

  Insulin (long-term storage)

  Hematopoietic agents such as Neupogen and Epogen

  Vaccines such as hepatitis A and B, tetanus, pneumococcal, and polio

  Tuberculin skin tests

  Antibiotic injectables that are ready to use, such as BiCillin LA and CR

  Suppositories such as Phenergan

  Tablets such as Volmax, Alkeran, and several new antiviral medications

  Oral liquids such as EES ready-to-use suspension and Orapred

  Some ophthalmic preparations such as Viroptic solution

  Controlled substances such as Ativan injection

- Freezer (less than 32°F or 0°C)

Each refrigerator should have its own temperature records, and personnel in each department should check the temperature of the refrigerator at least daily. This daily check should be documented in writing and initialed by the responsible personnel.

Safe Handling of Cytotoxic and Hazardous Materials

Cytotoxic and hazardous materials used in the pharmacy require special handling to preserve the safety of both the product and the personnel. The federal Occupational Safety and Health Administration (OSHA) sets standards that govern the special handling and storage of cytotoxic, antineoplastic, or chemotherapy agents as well as other chemicals such as bleach, alcohol, and acids.

OSHA defines a hazardous agent as one that could be either a health hazard or a physical hazard. If there is evidence that either acute or chronic health effects could result if personnel were exposed to the chemical itself, then it should be considered hazardous. Some agents in this category are

- Carcinogens
- Toxins
- Irritants
- Corrosives
- Other agents that could damage the lungs, eyes, ears, skin, or mucous membranes

A physical hazard is one that could cause physical damage in the workplace. Examples of these types of chemicals are

- Combustible liquids
- Compressed gases
- Explosives
- Flammables

OSHA standards require that personnel who may be exposed to potentially dangerous drugs and chemicals must complete an orientation and training process that covers all policies and procedures followed by the facility. Personnel should receive "Worker Right to Know" information with this orientation and training.

OSHA requires documentation such as Material Safety Data Sheets (MSDS) for all hazardous materials and chemicals to be stored in the pharmacy. Along with the MSDS, proper warning labels to identify hazardous chemicals are also required.

The MSDS are designed to inform personnel (both employees and emergency responders) about proper procedures for handling a particular substance. These sheets are not meant for consumers but for those who work around and with these chemicals and other hazardous substances on a day-to-day basis. The MSDS should be kept readily available and easily accessible to anyone who may need them at any time. Generally, a binder is kept on the premises that contains MSDS for all chemicals and other hazardous substances that are used or stored in the area. As new items become part of the pharmacy inventory, an MSDS should accompany their arrival and become part of the MSDS file on hand.

The MSDS include information on:

- Chemical name and Chemical Abstract Service (CAS) number
- Flammability
- Reactivity
- Flash point
- Department of Transportation (DOT) warnings
- Stability
- National Fire Protection Association (NFPA) classification

Some physical data about the chemical is also listed on the MSDS, including:

- Boiling point
- Specific gravity
- Melting point
- Vapor pressure and density

Storage areas for these products should be designed to prevent damage, breakage, spillage, or leakage. Bins and shelves should have frontal barriers to prevent containers from dropping to the floor and breaking or spilling. Hazardous medications to be stored under refrigeration must be kept separate from other medications. They also should be kept in a fashion designed to prevent breakage and contain leakage should a break occur. Hazardous drugs should never be placed in dumbwaiters or pneumatic tubes for transport because mechanical stress on the product could result in contamination of all the areas involved.

As a precaution, pregnant women should not handle cytotoxic or hazardous agents. However, even though dangers and hazardous substances are used and stored within the area where you work, the pharmacy workplace does not have to be hazardous to your health. Safety should be everyone's concern, and all personnel should have the proper training to ensure that the work area is safe for all. Additional industry guidelines and recommendations for handling/preparing hazardous drugs have been established by the National Institute for Occupational Safety and Health (NIOSH), the American Society of Health-System Pharmacists (ASHP) and the International Society of Oncology Pharmacy Practitioners (ISOPP).

Medication Distribution

In an inpatient facility, the pharmacy department is in control and is responsible for all the medication throughout the facility. Medication distribution areas includes the unit-dose area, floor stock, and IV admixtures.

When a medication order is received by the pharmacy, it is entered into the computer and the pharmacy technician fills the order in the unit-dose area. In the pharmacy's unit-dose area, all medications are individually packaged, and most packages contain one unit of medication. Unit-dose packages are individually labeled with the drug name, strength, dosage form, lot number, expiration date, and manufacturer. The technician fills medications for each new order as they arrive and for the entire patient population during patient cassette fill. In retail pharmacies, most routine and maintenance prescriptions are dispensed in supplies of 30 days or more. In a hospital pharmacy, patient medications are generally dispensed in 24-hour increments. This means that the pharmacy fills all the medications needed for each patient every 24 hours using unit-dose medications.

Medication distribution in an inpatient facility includes more than just delivering patient-specific medication to the appropriate area. In a hospital, non–patient-specific medication is also distributed by the pharmacy. This type of medication includes floor stock, emergency medications in crash/code carts, and medications stored in automated dispensing systems and after-hours or night cabinets.

Floor Stock

Floor stock medications are drugs that are kept outside the pharmacy and are not intended specifically for any one patient. When one of these medications is needed, it can be retrieved from floor stock instead of getting it from the pharmacy. Although these medications are stored outside the pharmacy, the pharmacy is still responsible for the storage, control, processing, and billing of floor stock medications.

In the past, floor stock medications were usually controlled substances, stat or PRN drugs, and emergency drugs, because all routine drugs were dispensed from the pharmacy. However, with automated dispensing technology, many floor stock systems now include routine medications as well. When a floor stock system is automated and includes routine medications, it reduces the amount of medication that are dispensed specifically for each individual patient. Drugs included in an institution's floor stock vary from institution to institution.

Automated Dispensing Systems

The profession of pharmacy has gradually evolved into providing pharmaceutical care. Changes that occurred during this evolution have caused health care systems to seek cost-reducing measures and more effective patient/medication safety. As a result, automated dispensing systems and devices are common in today's pharmacies.

The purpose of automation is to enhance patient care and relieve the pharmacist from some of the medication distribution process. Pharmacy technicians are the primary personnel involved in working with, maintaining, and stocking automated dispensing systems. Automated devices such as Pyxis, Omnicell, MedCarousel, and Acu-Dose are used in hospital settings. ScriptPro and Parata are automated dispensing systems used in retail pharmacies. The manufacturers of these different systems also produce accompanying software that can be interfaced with the existing pharmacy software, which makes it much easier to adapt to the new technologies.

Automated systems are intended for use in the distribution of both individual patient prescriptions in retail and unit-dose medication orders in hospitals.

Some specific features of hospital automated dispensing systems include the following.

- Medications are contained and administered from unit-dose packaging.
- Medications are provided or dispensed in ready-to-use form when possible.
- Medication is accessible only at the time it is to be administered for patient use.
- A profile of all medications concurrently being used is maintained in pharmacy records for each specific patient.

Crash or Code Carts

A crash or code cart is a wheeled cart that contains the medication, equipment, and supplies that must be readily available for patient resuscitation during cardiac arrest and other medical emergencies. Medical facilities have crash carts in all patient care areas. When a patient stops breathing, goes into cardiac arrest, or otherwise "crashes," a

"Code Blue" is called and the medical personnel wheel the cart to the patient and begin resuscitative measures.

Because the crash cart contains medication, the pharmacy is responsible for ensuring that the proper medication is included on the cart. This includes making sure all required medications are present, that no drugs are expired, and checking for package integrity. Medication can be included on the cart in trays that fit inside the drawers or in tackle boxes that sit on top of the cart.

The pharmacy is responsible for maintaining crash cart drugs and IV solutions, and the technician is responsible for its inventory. All other equipment and supplies are the responsibility of the respective departments. Technicians conduct crash cart inventories during their monthly nursing station inspections or after the crash cart has been used. In most facilities, after the crash cart is opened or used, the medication trays or boxes are brought to the pharmacy and exchanged for new, sealed trays. In other facilities, the technician must go to the patient care area to inventory the medication and replace or exchange any drug that has been used or has expired. All medication replaced or exchanged in a crash cart must be checked by the pharmacist.

Most drugs carried in crash carts are in injectable form. Because these drugs must be administered quickly, many are available in prefilled syringes (PFS). Prefilled syringes do not require personnel to spend precious time opening syringes and needles and drawing up medications.

Compounding and Repackaging of Pharmaceuticals

Compounding is a very important part of pharmacy practice. Sometimes a patient's need for a unique dosage form requires pharmacy personnel to provide medications in forms that are not available commercially. Compounding can either be extemporaneous—preparing medication for a specific patient—or bulk—preparing medication in anticipation of a prescription.

Compounding in the pharmacy should be performed in compliance with specific guidelines set forth in the pharmacy's policies and procedures manual. Each part of the process should also be done in accordance with all applicable state and federal laws governing compounding. Good record-keeping is imperative to ensure the quality of the finished product, which in turn affects the quality of care available to the patient.

A master formula should be on file for every product compounded in the pharmacy. This master formula is a set of specific instructions for making the product. It includes a listing of all materials, equipment, and supplies needed to produce a certain quantity, weight, or volume of the compounded product. The master formula should include the following information:

- Product name
- Dosage form
- Specifications and/or sources of raw materials
- Weights and measures of each raw material
- Total quantity, volume, or weight yielded
- Equipment needed
- Shelf-life and expiration-date considerations
- Packaging and storage requirements
- Sample label and auxiliary labels
- Step-by-step instructions for the entire compounding process
- Quality-control testing measures, if any
- References or source of the formula, if possible

For each bulk compounded product, exact production records should be kept. A production log should be maintained so that records will be readily available if they are ever needed. The production log should include, but not be limited to, the following information:

- Date of compounding
- Lot or batch number assigned
- Manufacturer's lot number and name for each raw material used in the compound
- Weights and measures performed
- A statement of final yield
- Final verification signatures
- Sample labeling
- Product expiration date
- Mechanism of verification for both the person compounding and the person verifying

The log should be kept on file for the length of time specified under all applicable laws. This is generally one year past the product's expiration date.

Correct product labeling is as important as any other part of the compounding process. The label should be permanent and contain the following:

- Product name and strength
- Dosage form
- Lot or batch number
- Storage conditions
- Expiration date
- Any auxiliary labels or other special instructions needed
- Any other information required by law

Because the packaging helps maintain the stability and quality of the product, it should be appropriate for the dosage form. For instance, suppositories should be wrapped and placed in boxes, and ointments and creams should be packed in jars or tubes made for their storage. Elixirs, syrups, and suspensions should be kept in calibrated bottles intended for storing liquid medications. Sterile compounded products should be kept in packaging that is sterile and free of particulate matter. The packaging should protect from light and moisture to preserve shelf life.

The pharmacy technician must follow written procedures for each specific compound. The pharmacist must perform quality checks and verifications at appropriate critical points in the process to ensure that the end result will meet the specifications for that product.

The area used for compounding should be sanitary. Work surfaces should permit effective cleaning to minimize the potential for contamination, and the entire area should be conducive to an orderly workflow to minimize the risk of adding any extraneous materials to the product.

Technicians are responsible for the proper care, function, and maintenance of compounding equipment. Equipment must be used safely and only for its intended use, and it must be cleaned properly to reduce contamination risks. Quality-assurance measures should be taken to ensure that all preventive maintenance procedures are followed, and periodic checks should be made to ensure proper function and correct calibration.

Not only do the equipment and work areas need to maintain a high level of cleanliness, all personnel involved in the compounding process should follow strict personal hygiene guidelines. When compounding a nonsterile medication, pharmacy technicians should always wash their hands properly, to prevent contamination of the product and to protect themselves. Hands should be washed up to the elbows.

The compounder's head, hands, face, and arms should be covered by attire that is appropriate to perform his or her duties properly. What is considered proper attire will depend on the product being compounded and the pharmacy's policies and procedures.

At a minimum, technicians should wear a clean lab coat and gloves for most nonsterile compounding. Written guidelines documented in the policies and procedures manual should be followed for quality assurance of the compounded product and safety of both the technician and the patient.

Repackaging Oral Solids and Liquids

When a unit-dose package is not available, too expensive to purchase, or a special dose or package is needed, the pharmacy will repackage those drugs from bulk containers into individual unit-dose packages. Repackaging is a primary responsibility of the pharmacy technician.

When repackaging, pharmacy technicians should:

- Not repackage more than one drug product at a time and should not have any other labels than those used for the present repackaging processes in the immediate area, in order to avoid mislabeling or cross-contamination of drug products.
- Remove all remaining medications and labels when repackaging is completed. Furthermore, equipment and work areas should be left empty, clean, and ready for the next operation run.
- Use all packaging equipment and printing devices only in the manner intended by the manufacturer of those products. Any deviation from those intended uses must be justified and approved by the pharmacy supervisor.

The following American Society of Health-System Pharmacists (ASHP) guidelines for packages, personnel, facilities, equipment, labels, records, and storage should be followed when repackaging medications.

Packages

Unit-dose packages must:

- Identify the contents of the container completely and precisely.
- Protect the contents from harmful environmental effects such as light and moisture.
- Protect the contents from breakage and contamination that may be caused by handling.
- Permit the contents to be used in a quick, easy, and safe manner.

Containers and closures are classified according to the degree to which contents are protected. The four types of containers are

1. Light-resistant
2. Well closed (protects from extraneous solids and from loss of drug under normal circumstances)
3. Tight (protects from extraneous solids, liquids, and vapors and from evaporation, melting, or loss of drug under normal circumstances)
4. Hermetic (impervious to air or any other gases under ordinary conditions)

Personnel

A quality-check person (pharmacist) must approve or reject all repackaging.

Protective Apparel

Personnel should wear protective clothing as necessary to protect drug products from contamination. At a minimum, gloves and a clean lab coat should be worn.

Facilities

Each pharmacy that performs repackaging activities must have a separate area that is well lighted, ventilated, and has the proper temperature control.

Equipment

Repackaging equipment should be kept clean and in proper working order at all times and should be kept off the floor to prevent contamination.

Labels

Labels are to be typewritten or computer generated. Each label must include the drug's brand name, strength, and dosage form or generic name, strength, dosage form, and manufacturer, the quantity of the drug if the quantity if greater than 1 unit, the facility's unique lot number, and an expiration date based on current literature. Technicians should take extra care when preparing labels, as this is the most common source of errors.

Records

Repackaging labels should include name of drug, strength, dosage form, facility lot number, manufacturer, manufacturer's lot number and expiration date, facility's expiration date, quantity per repackaged unit, number of repackaged units prepared, date packaged, and name, initials, or electronic signature of repackager and verifying pharmacist.

Storage

All repackaged products, stock containers, and records must be quarantined in an area where there is no chance of their being used until they are checked and released by the pharmacist.

SUMMARY

Pharmacy technicians play a crucial role in the control of inventory and maintenance of stocked medications, regardless of the practice setting. It is important to understand these concepts, not only for the national certification exam, but to be a successful and competent working pharmacy technician.

CHAPTER REVIEW QUESTIONS

1. When using an order-point system for inventory control, which of the following statements are true?
   a. As inventoried items are used during the filling process, the inventory levels of each item are automatically reduced and tallied.
   b. When an item's inventory level drops below the minimum level, it reaches the order point.
   c. Upon reaching its order point, a particular item is automatically placed on the next order with the wholesaler.
   d. all of the above

2. Medications used in emergency situations are
   a. available on the crash cart
   b. available mostly in prefilled syringes
   c. inventoried, stocked, and delivered by the pharmacy technician
   d. all the above

3. All of the following agencies receive a copy of DEA Form 222 except:
   a. the DEA
   b. the FDA
   c. the pharmacy
   d. the wholesaler or supplier

4. What is the correct temperature for storing an item under refrigeration?
   a. 59–86°F
   b. 46–59°F
   c. 36–46°F
   d. 32–36°F

5. Which organization requires that MSDS be kept on file for all hazardous materials and chemicals stored in the pharmacy?
   a. Joint Commission
   b. OSHA
   c. DEA
   d. FDA
   e. ASHP

6. Which of the following areas contains patient-specific medications?
   a. unit-dose carts
   b. nursing floor stock
   c. emergency crash carts
   d. automated dispensing systems

7. Of the following drugs, which is not classified as a Schedule II drug?
   a. oxycodone (Percocet, Tylox)
   b. methylphenidate (Concerta, Ritalin)
   c. hydroxychloroquine (Plaquenil)
   d. fentanyl (Sublimaze)

8. Of all FDA recalls, which is the least likely to cause serious adverse health consequences?
   a. Class I
   b. Class II
   c. Class III
   d. Class IV

9. Where can guidelines governing compounding specific to each pharmacy be found?
   a. compounding supply catalog
   b. policies and procedures manual
   c. MSDS
   d. U.S. Pharmacopeia

10. A set of specific instructions for making each product compounded in the pharmacy, including lists of all materials, equipment, and supplies needed, is known as:
   a. a production log
   b. a repackaging log
   c. a master formula
   d. none of the above

chapter 4

Participating in the Administration and Management of Pharmacy Practice

After completing this chapter, you should be able to:

* List the specific competencies pertaining to administration and management of pharmacy practice that are covered on the certification exam.

* List the specific knowledge and skills required for pharmacy technicians to participate effectively in the administration and management of pharmacy practice.

* Explain the administration and management of pharmacy practice as it relates to various practice settings.

* Define basic business terms and concepts as they relate to pharmacy practice.

Introduction

The third section of the Pharmacy Technician Certification Examination (PTCE), titled "Participating in the Administration and Management of Pharmacy Practice," comprises 12% of the exam. The content includes the following:

■ Coordinate written, electronic, and oral communications throughout the practice setting (for example, route phone calls, faxes, verbal and written refill authorizations; disseminate policy changes).

■ Update and maintain information (for example, insurance information, patient demographics, provider information, reference material).

■ Collect productivity information (for example, the number of prescriptions filled, fill times, money collected, rejected-claim status).

■ Participate in quality-improvement activities (for example, medication error reports, customer satisfaction surveys, delivery audits, internal audits of processes).

- Generate quality-assurance reports.
- Implement and monitor the practice setting for compliance with federal, state, and local laws, regulations, and professional standards (for example, Material Safety Data Sheets [MSDS], eyewash centers, Joint Commission [formerly known as JCAHO] standards).
- Implement and monitor policies and procedures for sanitation management, handling of hazardous waste (for example, needles), and infection control (for example, protective clothing, laminar airflow hood, other equipment cleaning).
- Perform and record routine sanitation, maintenance, and calibration of equipment (for example, automated dispensing equipment, balances, robotics, refrigerator temperatures).
- Maintain and use manual or computer-based information systems to perform job-related activities (for example, update prices, generate reports and labels, perform utilization tracking and inventory control).
- Maintain software for automated dispensing technology, including point-of-care drug-dispensing cabinets.
- Perform billing and accounting functions (for example, personal charge accounts, third-party rejections, third-party reconciliation, census maintenance, prior authorization).
- Communicate with third-party payers to determine or verify coverage.
- Conduct staff training.
- Aid in establishing, implementing, and monitoring policies and procedures.

Knowledge

The knowledge base required to perform activities associated with the third section of the PTCE includes the following knowledge areas:

- The practice setting's mission, goals and objectives, organizational structure, and policies and procedures
- Lines of communication throughout the organization
- Principles of resource allocation (for example, scheduling, cross training, work flow)
- Productivity, efficiency, and customer satisfaction measures
- Written, oral, and electronic communication systems
- Required operational licenses and certificates
- Roles and responsibilities of pharmacists, pharmacy technicians, and other pharmacy employees

- Legal and regulatory requirements for personnel, facilities, equipment, and supplies (for example, space requirements, prescription file storage, cleanliness, reference materials, storage of radiopharmaceuticals)
- Professional standards (for example, the Joint Commission) for personnel, facilities, equipment, and supplies
- Quality-improvement standards and guidelines
- State pharmacy board regulations
- Storage requirements and expiration dates for equipment and supplies (for example, first-aid items, fire extinguishers)
- Storage and handling requirements for hazardous substances (for example, chemotherapeutics, radiopharmaceuticals)
- Hazardous-waste disposal requirements
- Procedures for treatment of exposure to hazardous substances (for example, eyewash)
- Security systems for the protection of employees, customers, and property
- Laminar airflow hood maintenance requirements
- Infection-control policies and procedures
- Sanitation requirements (for example, hand washing and cleaning counting trays, countertops, and equipment)
- Equipment calibration and maintenance procedures
- Procurement procedures for supplies
- Technology used in the preparation, delivery, and administration of medications (for example, robotics, Baker cells, automated total parenteral nutrition [TPN] equipment, Pyxis, infusion pumps)
- Purpose and function of pharmacy equipment
- Documentation requirements for routine sanitation, maintenance, and equipment calibration
- Americans with Disabilities Act (ADA) requirements (for example, physical accessibility)
- Manual and computer-based systems for storing, retrieving, and using pharmacy information (for example, drug interactions, patient profiles, generation of labels)
- Security procedures related to data integrity, security, and confidentiality
- Downtime emergency policies and procedures
- Backup and archiving procedures for stored data and documentation
- Legal requirements regarding archiving
- Third-party reimbursement systems
- Health care reimbursement systems (for example, home health, respiratory medications, eligibility, and reimbursement)
- Billing and accounting policies and procedures
- Information sources used to obtain data in a quality-improvement system (for example, the patient's chart, patient profile, computerized information systems, medication administration record)
- Procedures to document occurrences such as medication errors, adverse effects, and product integrity (for example, the Food and Drug Administration [FDA] MedWatch program)
- Staff training techniques
- Employee performance evaluation techniques
- Employee performance feedback techniques

Skills

A pharmacy technician should be able to do the following:

- Communicate clearly, both orally and in writing, with professional staff, manufacturers' representatives, and distributors.
  - Organize all written or verbal communication logically.
  - Address all communications at an appropriate level.
  - Use correct grammar, punctuation, spelling, style, and formatting conventions in the preparation of all written communications.
  - Pronounce technical terms correctly.
  - Use listening skills consistently in the performance of job functions.
- Use computers to perform pharmacy functions related to inventory control, ordering, and stock status reports.
  - Explain the typical database used to support pharmacy management functions.
  - Demonstrate ability to order by bar code.
  - Demonstrate ability to order by computer modem.
  - Demonstrate ability to order by fax.
- Purchase pharmaceutical devices and supplies according to an established purchasing program.
  - Describe typical procedures for purchasing pharmaceutical devices, and describe typical procedures used to expedite emergency orders.
  - Demonstrate the ability to follow established procedures for ordering medications.
- Identify pharmaceuticals, durable medical equipment, devices, and supplies to be ordered.
  - Explain the importance of maintaining an adequate supply of pharmaceuticals.
  - Explain the role that judgment plays in supplementing an automated system for determining the timing and amount of pharmaceuticals, durable medical equipment, devices, and supplies to order.
- Explain alternative strategies for securing a pharmacy item that is not available.
  - State categories of alternative sources of items not available from the primary vendor at time of need.
  - Explain the importance of evaluating the costs of securing a needed item from an alternative source.
  - Explain acceptable methods for communicating changes in product availability to patients, caregivers, and/or health care professionals.
- Control the inventory of medications, equipment, and devices according to an established plan.
  - Describe the various methods of inventory control.
  - Follow established policies and procedures for receiving goods and verifying specification on the original order.
  - Describe the general tasks involved in receiving and verifying the order of goods.
  - Describe methods for handling back-ordered medications.
- Follow established policies and procedures to maintain a record of controlled substances received, stored, and removed from inventory.
  - State the legal requirements for recording controlled substances received.
  - State the procedure for destroying controlled substances.
  - Demonstrate the ability to maintain an inventory of controlled substances.

- Follow established policies and procedures for removing from inventory expired or discontinued pharmaceuticals, durable medical equipment, devices, supplies, or recalled items in these same categories.
  - Define the terms *expired, discontinued,* and *recalled* as used in pharmacy.
  - Describe common reasons for discontinuing or recalling items.
  - Explain the role of documenting item removal in maintaining an inventory system.
  - Explain the importance of maintaining a record of prepacking, recalls, and returns of pharmaceuticals, durable medical equipment, devices, and supplies.
  - Demonstrate the ability to follow established procedures for removing items from inventory.
- Demonstrate the ability to manage the institutional formulary.
  - Explain the federal and state laws governing the substitution of drug products.
  - Explain the purpose and use of a formulary.
  - Explain the influence that the formulary and/or policies of third-party payers have on the selection of products.
  - Explain the procedure for addition or removal of a drug from a formulary.
  - Follow an established program to collect data efficiently and accurately for use by the pharmacists in managing pharmacy services.
  - State the types of information that pharmacists might request to assist in managing pharmacy services.

Pharmacy Practice

Whether technicians work in retail or institutional pharmacies, they have to be skilled in the administration and management of pharmacy practice in their setting. A major skill needed in both setting is good communication skills. Technicians must be able to understand and be understood to avoid pharmacy errors. Although technicians in a retail setting communicate primarily with patients and technicians in an institutional setting communicate primarily with health care professionals, the skills needed for good communication are the same.

Communication skills are vital to the delivery of pharmaceutical care in all pharmacy settings. A skilled pharmacy technician must be able to communicate with other trained health professionals and at the same time be able to communicate effectively with patients who have little or no knowledge about their prescriptions.

Think of communication as a two-way street. Effective communication involves understanding the exchange of information between the patient or health professional and the technician. Communicating properly takes effort, and it is just as important to listen and understand what someone is saying as it is to impart or disseminate information.

Although listening is sometimes considered a passive activity, to understand properly what is being said, a person must be actively involved in listening. This is important because not all communication is verbal. Nonverbal forms of communication, such as body language, which includes facial expressions, posture, hand motions, eye contact, and physical proximity, are valuable communication indicators to the listener. Voice tone and pitch are also important components. For example, you may ask a patient how he is doing and he may answer "Just fine," but you can tell by his body language and expression that he is not "just fine."

A good communicator is also aware of communication barriers that may inhibit the message from being fully understood. Communication barriers can include physical or emotional impairments as well cultural and language differences. A skilled technician must be able to recognize these barriers and accommodate them.

An excellent technique for technicians to ensure that patients comprehend them is to ask open-ended questions. For example, after you have given a patient detailed instructions, ask her to tell you how she is going to take a medication. A simple smile or nod of the head does not indicate understanding, but repeating instructions back correctly does indicate comprehension.

Cultural and language differences can also be barriers to effective communication. One culture may find things such as eye contact or standing within 18 inches of another person uncomfortable. Patients from some cultures may be offended if you address them by their first name. Although English is the most-used language in the United States, many patients have another language as their native language. As an English-speaking technician, you must be aware of language differences that may cause miscommunication and medication errors. For example, *once* in English means "one time," whereas in Spanish it is the number 11. Think of how often we use *once* in our directions to patients. What would be the difference if they hear it as "eleven"?

The Business of Pharmacy

For any business to succeed, it must operate in such a manner that the revenue (the money coming into the business) exceeds the expenses (the money that it costs to do business). Every employee is an important part of this process. Pharmacists and technicians must provide pharmaceutical care for their patients while managing the business in a profitable manner.

Because the bottom line in any business, including pharmacy, is profit, it is important for pharmacy technicians to understand some basic business concepts. To realize a profit, a business must take in more through sales than its expenses. Remember that if the pharmacy is making money, the technicians' job security is greater. However, if the pharmacy is not turning a profit, everyone's job may be in jeopardy.

In an expansion of typical duties, many technicians are becoming more and more involved in the business end of pharmacy. Following are some business terms and concepts it is important for technicians to know.

Accounts payable ledger A record of what a pharmacy owes its suppliers and other creditors.

Accounts receivable ledger A record of what is owed to the pharmacy by patients, insurance companies, government agencies, and managed-care contractors.

Asset Anything that is owned by the pharmacy.

Average wholesale price (AWP) The average price at which a wholesaler sells a drug to pharmacies.

Balance sheet A statement of the financial condition of the business at a given time, which uses the basic equation, assets = liabilities + net worth.

Capitation A fixed fee paid to a pharmacy by an insurance company to provide medications to a patient. The pharmacy does not get additional fees if the patient's prescriptions cost more that what has been reimbursed. Likewise, the insurance company does not receive any money back if the costs of the prescriptions are less than the fixed fee paid.

Cash disbursements journal A record of pharmacy expenditures.

Cash flow statement A record of cash receipts and disbursements.

Cash receipts journal A record of cash that comes into the business.

General journal A book that contains all business activities.

Income statement A record of profit or loss that shows the financial transactions that have occurred over a specified time period.

Inventory A record of the business's investment in merchandise and equipment.

Invoice A document showing items purchased at one time from a specific supplier.

Liability What is owed to a creditor.

Maximum allowable cost (MAC) The maximum amount a pharmacy will be reimbursed for a prescription drug.

Net worth The value of the business that belongs to the owner.

Overhead The ongoing cost of running the business. Overhead includes utilities, rent, and so on.

Purchase journal A record of purchases of merchandise for resale.

Sales journal A record that summarizes monthly revenues.

Accounting records must be kept for tax purposes as well as for general business use. Pharmacies use a variety of systems to record financial items. Some pharmacies contract with accounting agencies; others have an in-house employee keep the books. No matter which method is used, it is important to maintain current, accurate financial records using a process that is flexible, easily understood, inexpensive, not time-intensive, and convenient to use.

Product pricing is important to the success of the business of pharmacy. Most non-prescription items are priced based on a percentage markup. Different markup values are often used for different product categories. For example, a 1-ounce tube of antibiotic ointment may be marked up 40%. If the tube costs the pharmacy $1.40, then 40% of the cost will be added to obtain the selling price. The formula for calculating markup is

$$selling\ price = cost + (cost \times markup)$$
$$selling\ price = \$1.40 + \$1.40 * 0.402$$
$$= \$1.40 + \$0.562$$
$$= \$1.96$$

The markup on costume jewelry may be 100%. For example, a necklace may cost the pharmacy $10.00. We would add 100% of the cost back to the cost to obtain the selling price:

$$selling\ price = \$10.00 + \$10.00 * 1.02$$
$$= \$10.00 + 10.00$$
$$= \$20.00$$

However, $19.95 sounds less expensive than $20.00, so let's sell the necklace for $19.95. Most retail prices traditionally end in either 5 or 9.

Another management aspect of pharmacy as a business is advertising. The best business in the world must still reach its potential customers. Pharmacies use various advertising media: television, radio, billboards, direct mailings, newspaper ads, and Internet banner ads. Pharmacy owners or managers should determine a budget for advertising. Characteristics of the customer base are important factors when developing an advertising plan. In some communities, an ad in the program for the local high school football team may be more productive than one in other media. However, the most effective advertising is the word of mouth of a satisfied customer. The physical location and the layout of a pharmacy are also important factors. Traffic flow should be considered before establishing a pharmacy. Easy access and generous parking are advantages. Drive-through service may be an added bonus for certain customers. The mom with several children in the vehicle and the elderly lady with arthritis may choose a particular pharmacy because of the drive-through. Customer flow within the pharmacy also needs to be considered. Most retail pharmacies have the prescription department in the back of the store. This placement is intentional, because the "business" hopes that customers will make additional purchases as they walk through the rest of the store to reach the prescription counter.

Work flow within the pharmacy department should be designed for efficiency. Pharmacy technicians and pharmacists need to have everything positioned in the pharmacy so that the actual dispensing process proceeds from the input area to the patient counseling area without crossover traffic or interference. Locations of telephones, computers, and printers are important, as is the placement of automated dispensing devices, which require large amounts of space. All aspects of the dispensing process should be carefully considered to determine the most efficient use of pharmacy department space and to ensure that prescriptions are filled quickly and accurately.

Policies and Procedures

The practice of pharmacy has changed vastly over the past decades as a result of new drugs, delivery systems, automation, government regulations, and the growth of professional organizations. The American Society of Health-System Pharmacists (ASHP) was one of the first organizations to develop standards of practice for hospital pharmacy.

Today, the ASHP minimum standards state: "An operations manual governing pharmacy functions (e.g., administrative, operational, and clinical) shall exist."

All pharmacies are required to have written policies and procedures (P&Ps) for all pharmacy-related operations. These written documents are gathered together in one book or manual called a policy and procedures manual. This manual should contain all applicable P&Ps as well as long-term goals for the pharmacy.

P&Ps are not just for the pharmacy. Every department in the institution or organization will have P&Ps specific to their operations and departmental needs. There will also be an institutional or organizational policy and procedures manual. Departmental policies and procedures should not conflict with the organization's P&Ps.

Policies and procedures are also sometimes referred to as standards of practice (SOPs), and these two terms may be used interchangeably. Pharmacy technicians must be familiar with the P&Ps or SOPs of their respective pharmacies: Their job depends on it.

A *policy* can be defined as "a definite course or method of action selected from among alternatives and in light of given conditions to guide and determine present and future decisions." Policies are written statements that provide a framework for action and are considered broad guidelines for the pharmacy. An example of a policy is

Pharmacy Conduct, Behavior, and Appearance

The Pharmacy Department, due to the nature of its responsibilities and functions, shall have strict standards of employee conduct and behavior.

A *procedure* can be defined as "a particular way of accomplishing something or of acting; a statement of a series of systems to implement the policies of the department or organization." A procedure is a written instruction that describes the sequential steps necessary to complete a specific task. An example of a procedure is

---

PROCEDURE

1. Conduct

a. All Pharmacy Department employees are to conduct themselves in a courteous and professional manner at all times.

b. When dealing with the public or with other hospital employees, each employee is a representative of the entire Pharmacy Department and the institution. A helpful and polite manner shall be maintained at all times. Conditions and situation that could lead to potential conflicts or disagreements should be referred to a supervisor.

Besides being required, a well-written policy and procedures manual has many benefits, including that it:

1. Improves both inter- and intradepartmental communication
2. Creates standards of care
3. Provides a mechanism for documenting standards of care
4. Enhances staff orientation and training
5. Improves and maintains staff morale
6. Enables management to systematically, objectively, and efficiently measure staff and departmental performance
7. Provides a source of information
8. Encourages cost-effective use of resources
9. Provides an administrative tool for planning, developing, and improving pharmacy service

The manual should contain information telling employees how to perform day-to-day tasks as well as the procedure to follow in case of emergencies. It should provide guidelines covering the responsibilities of each employee position as well as specifying the chain of command of employees. The policies and procedures manual should be created when the business is formed and should be updated on a regular basis.

Institutional pharmacies have a *pharmacy and therapeutics (P&T) committee,* which consists of pharmacy personnel and other institutional staff. The main responsibility of the P&T committee is to create and maintain the drug formulary, but it can also play an important role in developing P&Ps. Because the practice of pharmacy is constantly evolving, the formulary and P&Ps must be updated frequently.

An additional responsibility of the P&T committee is to implement these changes by notifying the staff to ensure that everyone stays current with respect to developments in pharmaceuticals. This may be accomplished by seminars, bulletins, and newsletters. The committee also provides a means for drug-use evaluation, medication-error reporting, and adverse-reaction reporting.

SUMMARY

Pharmaceutical care for the patient is the ultimate goal of all pharmacy services, no matter the location, the business plan, or the profit margin. All pharmacy personnel should remind themselves daily that pharmaceutical care is the responsible provision of drug therapy for the purpose of achieving definite outcomes that improve a patient's quality of life.

CHAPTER REVIEW QUESTIONS

1. A statement of the financial condition at a given time that uses the basic equation, assets = liabilities + net worth, is the:
   a. cash flow statement
   b. balance sheet
   c. income statement
   d. sales journal

2. Pharmacy advertising media include:
   a. television commercials
   b. radio ads
   c. direct mailings
   d. all of the above

3. Written guidelines stating directions for day-to-day tasks as well as the procedure to follow in case of emergencies are found in the:
   a. general journal
   b. policies and procedures manual
   c. employee handbook
   d. FDA handbook

4. The responsible provision of drug therapy for the purpose of achieving definite outcomes that improve a patient's quality of life is:
   a. prescription dispensing
   b. pharmaceutical care
   c. merchandising
   d. drug-utilization review

5. Nonverbal communication can include:
   a. facial expressions
   b. eye contact
   c. voice tone and pitch
   d. all of the above

6. The value of a business that belongs to the owner is the:
   a. liability
   b. asset
   c. net worth
   d. inventory

7. A record of profit or loss that shows the financial transactions that have occurred over a specified time period is the:
   a. income statement
   b. net worth
   c. sales journal
   d. balance sheet

8. The amount added to the cost of a product to calculate the selling price is the:
   a. rebate
   b. markup
   c. discount
   d. selling fee

9. A listing of medications that are approved to be prescribed and dispensed by a pharmacy institution is the:
   a. inventory
   b. invoice
   c. formulary
   d. dispensary

10. The pharmacy and therapeutics committee is responsible for all of the following except:
    a. drug-use evaluation
    b. medication-error reporting
    c. formulary revision
    d. maintenance of pharmacy inventory

chapter 5

Review of Pharmacy Calculations

LEARNING OBJECTIVES

After completing this chapter, you should be able to:

- Recognize and convert the various systems of measurement.
- Calculate ratios and proportions.
- Perform dosage calculations.
- Solve concentration and dilution problems.
- Calculate milliequivalents.
- Calculate flow rates.
- Solve alligations.
- Perform business calculations.

Introduction

Pharmacy calculations are often a large portion of the national pharmacy technician certification exams, and most students are very intimidated by math. However, it is imperative that pharmacy technicians be comfortable performing pharmacy calculations, because almost every aspect of pharmacy involves some sort of calculation. Therefore, to be successful on the certification exam and in practice, pharmacy technicians must master pharmaceutical calculations.

Systems of Measurement

As a pharmacy technician, you will rely on three systems of measurement to perform specific pharmacy calculations: the metric system, the household system, and the apothecary system. The metric system is the most widely recognized and utilized system for measurement in health care, but technicians must still be able to work with all three systems.

Tables 5-1 through 5-4 provide a review of the common metric prefixes and equivalents when working with the three systems of measurement.

Ratios and Proportions

Most pharmacy calculations can be solved using either an algebraic equation or using ratios and proportions. The ratio-and-proportion technique establishes two fractions that are equal to each other, using "given" and "needed" information in

Table 5-1 Metric System Prefixes with Standard Measures

	UNIT	ABBREVIATION	EQUIVALENTS
Weight	gram	g or gm	1 g = 1000 mg = 1,000,000 mcg
	milligram	mg	1 mg = 1000 mcg = 0.001 g
	microgram	mcg	1 mcg = 0.001 mg = 0.000001 g
	kilogram	kg	1 kg = 1000 g
Volume	liter	L or l	1 L = 1000 mL
	milliliter	mL or ml	1 mL = 1 cc = 0.001 L
	cubic centimeter	cc	1 cc = 1 mL = 0.001 L
Length	meter	m	1 m = 100 cm = 1000 mm
	centimeter	cm	1 cm = 0.01 m = 10 nm
	millimeter	mm	1 mm = 0.001 m = 0.1 cm

Table 5-2 Household Measure Equivalents

3 teaspoons	=	1 tablespoon
2 tablespoons	=	1 fluid ounce
8 fluid ounces	=	1 cup
2 cups	=	1 pint
2 pints	=	1 quart
4 quarts	=	1 gallon

Table 5-3 Household-to-Metric Conversions

HOUSEHOLD MEASURE		METRIC EQUIVALENT
1 teaspoon	=	5 mL
1 tablespoon	=	15 mL
1 fluid ounce	=	30 mL
1 pint	=	473 mL
1 gallon	=	3785 mL
1 cup	=	240 mL
1 ounce	=	28.35 g
1 pound	=	454 g
1 pound	=	16 oz

the problem. Once the ratios and proportions are determined, you can solve for the unknown x. When setting up ratios and proportions, determine what you "know" about the problem and set it equal to what is "needed or unknown," which is x. Always be sure that all units of measure are equivalent.

$$\text{what you know} = \text{what you need}$$
$$(\text{drug strength}) = (\text{patient dose})$$

Table 5-4 Apothecary-to-Metric Conversions

APOTHECARY MEASURE		METRIC EQUIVALENT
16.23 minims	=	1 mL
1 fluid dram	=	4 mL
1 fluid ounce	=	30 mL
1 ounce	=	8 drams
1 dram	=	60 grains
6 fluid ounces	=	180 mL
8 fluid ounces	=	240 mL
16 fluid ounces	=	500 mL
32 fluid ounces	=	1000 mL
1 grain	=	65 mg
1 ounce	=	480 grains
15 grains	=	1 g
1 pound	=	16 oz
2.2 pounds	=	1 kg

EXAMPLE: How much Amoxil, 250 mg/5 ml, should a patient take for each dose of the following prescription? Amoxicillin, 375 mg PO QID.

First, set up the problem. Be sure that all units of measure are the same on each side of the equation:

$$\text{what you know} = \text{what you need}$$
$$\frac{250 \text{ mg}}{5 \text{ ml}} = \frac{375 \text{ mg}}{x \text{ ml}}$$

Now, solve for x and cross-multiply:

$$250(x) = 375(5)$$
$$250x = 1875$$

Divide by 250 to get x by itself:

$$\frac{250x}{250} = \frac{1875}{250}$$
$$x = 7.5$$

Answer: $x = 7.5$ ml or 1½ tsp

Following are some examples of how ratios and proportions can be used in pharmacy calculations.

example **5.1**

Convert 2.5 oz to grams.

We know that $1 \text{ oz} = 30 \text{ g}$, so we can set up the following ratios and proportion:

$$\frac{1 \text{ oz}}{30 \text{ g}} = \frac{2.5 \text{ oz}}{x \text{ g}}$$

Cross-multiply and divide by x:

$$1x = 75$$
$$x = 75 \text{ g}$$

Answer: 2.5 oz is equivalent to 75 g.

====== IMPORTANT ======

Concentrations of many medications are expressed as a percent strength, such as Bactroban 2%. The percent strength represents how many grams of active ingredient are in 100 mL (liquid preparations) or 100 g (solid preparations). In other words, Bactroban 2% ointment would contain 2 g of drug per 100 g.

example 5.2

How many grams of drug are contained in 1 L of a 25% solution?

By definition, a 25% solution contains 25 g of drug per 100 mL; therefore, we can set up the following ratios and proportion:

$$\frac{25\,g}{100\ mL} = \frac{x}{1000\ mL}$$

Cross-multiply:

$$100x = 25,000$$

Divide both sides by 100:

$$\frac{100x}{100} = \frac{25,000}{100}$$
$$x = 250$$

Answer: $x = 250\,g$. Therefore, 1 L of a 25% solution contains 250 g of drug.

example 5.3

How many *milligrams* of drug are in 500 g of a 30% ointment?

By definition, a 30% ointment contains 30 g of drug per 100 g of ointment. Therefore, we can set up the following ratios and proportion:

$$\frac{30\,g}{100\,g} = \frac{x}{500\,g}$$

Cross-multiply:

$$100x = 15,000$$

Divide both sides by 100:

$$\frac{100x}{100} = \frac{15,000}{100}$$
$$x = 150$$

Answer: $x = 150\,g$. However, the question asked for *milligrams*, so the answer must be converted to milligrams:

$$\frac{1\,g}{150\,g} = \frac{1000\,mg}{x}$$

Cross-multiply:

$$1x = 150,000$$

Divide both sides by 1:

$$\frac{1x}{1} = \frac{150,000}{1}$$
$$x = 150,000$$

Thus, $x = 150,000$ mg Therefore, 500 g of a 30% ointment contains 150,000 mg of drug.

Dosage Calculations

Dosage calculations, which can include determining the number of doses, dispensing quantities, or ingredient quantities, are all performed using ratios and proportions.

example 5.4

Rx: Amoxicillin, 125 mg/5 mL, #150 mL, Sig: 1 tsp po tid. How many doses will be dispensed in all? What is the prescription days' supply?

We know that 1 tsp = 5 mL and that tid means three times per day; therefore, we can set up the following ratios and proportions:

$$\frac{1 \text{ tsp}}{5 \text{ mL}} = \frac{x \text{ tsp}}{150 \text{ mL}}$$

Cross-multiply:

$$5x = 150$$

Divide both sides by 5:

$$\frac{5x}{5} = \frac{150}{5}$$

Answer: $x = 30$ tsp. Therefore, this order contains 30 tsp, or 30 doses in total.

Next, how long will the prescription last if the patient takes the drug tid?

$$\frac{3 \text{ doses}}{1 \text{ day}} = \frac{30 \text{ doses}}{x \text{ days}}$$

Cross-multiply:

$$3x = 30$$

Divide both sides by 3:

$$\frac{3x}{3} = \frac{30}{3}$$

Answer: $x = 10$ days. Therefore, this order will last for 10 days.

example 5.5

Rx: Amoxicillin, 125 mg/5 mL, #150 mL, Sig: 1 tsp po tid. How many grams of amoxicillin is in 150 mL?

There are 125 mg per teaspoon, so we can set up the following ratios and proportion:

$$\frac{125 \text{ mg}}{5 \text{ mL}} = \frac{x}{150 \text{ mL}}$$

Cross-multiply:

$$5x = 18,750$$

Divide both sides by 5:

$$\frac{5x}{5} = \frac{18,750}{5}$$

$$x = 3750 \text{ mg}$$

Answer: Because $x = 3750$ mg, this order contains 3.75 g or 3750 mg of amoxicillin.

example 5.6

Rx: Hydroxyzine, 20 mg IV, q4–6h prn itching. How many milliliters of 25-mg/ml hydroxyzine is needed for each dose?

We know the drug strength is 25 mg/ml, and we need to know how many milliliters are needed for a 20-mg dose, so the proportion is

$$\frac{25\,mg}{ml} = \frac{20\,mg}{x\,ml}$$

Cross-multiply:

$$25(x) = 20(1)$$

Divide both sides by 25:

$$\frac{25x}{25} = \frac{20}{25}$$
$$x = 0.8$$

Answer: Because $x = 0.8$, we need 0.8 ml of 25-mg/ml hydroxyzine for a 20-mg dose.

Pediatric Dosing

Children and infants often require special considerations when calculating appropriate dosages. Common methods of calculating pediatric dosages are by body weight (mg/kg), by Fried's rule for infants, or by Clark's or Young's rule for children. When calculating by mg/kg, you will first need to convert the patient's weight from pounds to kilograms.

FORMULA

Weight Conversion

$$1\,kg = 2.2\,lb$$

Pediatric Dosing Based on Body Weight

example 5.7

A child weighs 45 lb; what is her weight in kilograms?

Using the weight conversion formula, you can set up the ratios and proportion:

$$\frac{1\,kg}{2.2\,lb} = \frac{x}{45\,lb}$$

Cross-multiply:

$$45 = 2.2x$$

Divide both sides by 2.2:

$$x = 20.45$$

This patient weighs 20.45 kg.

example 5.8

For the same patient as in Example 5.7, what is an appropriate dose for the following prescription? Rx: Ventolin syrup, 0.2 mg/kg/day in three divided doses.

Using the weight conversion from Example 5.7, set up the equation and solve:

$$0.2 \, \text{mg} \times 20.45 \, \text{kg} = 4.09$$

So this patient should receive 4.09 mg/day. Divide by 3 to calculate how much the patient will take for each dose; the answer is approximately 1.36 mg per dose.

example 5.9

Rx: Amoxicillin, 30 mg/kg/day divided q12h × 10 days. How much will the patient take with each dose, and how much should be dispensed for a 10-day supply? The drug available is amoxicillin, 125 mg/5 ml susp, and the patient weighs 27.5 lb.

First, convert weight the patient's weight from pounds to kilograms:

$$\frac{2.2 \, \text{lb}}{1 \, \text{kg}} = \frac{27.5 \, \text{lb}}{x \, \text{kg}}$$

Cross-multiply:

$$2.2(x) = 27.5(1)$$

Divide both sides by 2.2:

$$\frac{2.2x}{2.2} = \frac{27.5}{2.2}$$
$$x = 13.64$$

Answer: The patient's weight is 12.5 kg.

Next, you need 30 mg/kg per day divided q12h:

$$30 \, \text{mg} \times 12.5 \, \text{kg} = 375 \, \text{mg per day}$$
$$\frac{375 \, \text{mg}}{2 \, \text{doses per day}} = 187.5 \, \text{mg per dose}$$

Next, to determine how much should be given for each dose, set up a proportion:

$$\frac{125 \, \text{mg}}{5 \, \text{ml}} = \frac{187.5 \, \text{mg}}{x}$$

Cross-multiply:

$$125(x) = 187.5(5)$$

Divide both sides by 125:

$$\frac{125}{125} = \frac{937.5}{125}$$
$$x = 7.5$$

Answer: The patient dose is 7.5 ml.

To determine the amount to dispense for the prescription:

$$7.5 \, \text{ml} \times 2 \, \text{doses per day} \times 10 \, \text{days} = 150 \, \text{ml}$$

Pediatric Dosing Using Fried's, Clark's, and Young's Rules

FORMULA

Fried's Rule for Infants

$$\frac{\text{age (in months)} \times \text{adult dose}}{150} = \text{dose for infant}$$

example 5.10

The recommended adult dose for penicillin is 250 mg po q6h. What would the dose be for a nine-month-old infant?

Use Fried's rule:

$$\frac{9\,\text{months} \times 250\,\text{mg}}{150} = \text{infant's dose}$$

$$\text{infant's dose} = 15\,\text{mg}$$

Answer: The answer is 15 mg. Therefore, the penicillin dose for a nine-month-old infant is 15 mg every 6 hours.

FORMULA

Clark's Rule

$$\frac{\text{weight (pounds)} \times \text{adult dose}}{150} = \text{dose for child}$$

example 5.11

The recommended adult dose for erythromycin ethylsuccinate is 400 mg every 6 hours. What is the dose for a child who weighs 40 kg?

First, to use Clark's rule, the weight has to be in pounds, so convert 40 kg to pounds:

$$\frac{1\,\text{kg}}{2.2\,\text{lb}} = \frac{40\,\text{kg}}{x\,\text{lb}}$$

Cross-multiply:

$$2.2(40) = 1(x)$$

Divide both sides by 2.2:

$$\frac{40}{2.2} = \frac{1x}{2.2}$$

$$x = 88$$

Answer: The patient weighs 88 lb.

Now plug weight into the Clark's rule formula:

$$\frac{88 \times 400}{150} = \text{child's dose}$$

$$\frac{35{,}200}{150} = 234.666 \approx 234.67\,\text{mg}$$

Therefore, the dose for a child weighing 40 kg is 234.67 mg.

FORMULA

Young's Rule

$$\frac{\text{age (in years)} \times \text{adult dose}}{\text{age} + 12} = \text{dose for child}$$

---

example 5.12

The recommended adult dose for amoxicillin is 500 mg po q6h. What is the dose be for an eight-year-old child?

Use Young's rule:

$$\frac{8 \times 500 \text{ mg}}{8 + 12} = \text{child's dose}$$

$$\frac{4000}{20} = 200$$

Answer: The dose for an eight-year-old child is 200 mg.

Concentrations

Concentrations calculations are used to determine the percent strength or the amount of active ingredient in a particular preparation. *Percent* means parts per 100. The *percent strength* is the amount of the desired ingredient in the final product.

When solids are dissolved in liquids, the solid is considered the *solute* and the liquid is considered the *solvent*. When a liquid is mixed with another liquid, the liquid that occurs in the smaller quantity is the *solute* and the larger quantity of liquid is the *solvent*. Percentage concentrations of pharmaceuticals may be classified as one of the following three types:

$$\text{W/W\%} = \frac{\text{gm}}{100 \text{ gm}} = \text{number of grams of the drug in 100 gm of the final product}$$

$$\text{W/V\%} = \frac{\text{gm}}{100 \text{ ml}} = \text{number of grams of the drug in 100 ml of the final product}$$

$$\text{V/V\%} = \frac{\text{ml}}{100 \text{ ml}} = \text{number of milliliters of the drug in 100 ml of the final product}$$

EXAMPLES:

1. How many grams of dextrose are in 500 ml of D50W?
   D50W means that there are 50 gm of dextrose in 100 ml of final product.
   Therefore:

$$\frac{50 \text{ gm}}{100 \text{ ml}} = \frac{x \text{ gm}}{500 \text{ ml}} \rightarrow 100x = 50 \times 500 \rightarrow x = \frac{25,000}{100} \rightarrow x = 250 \text{ gm}$$

2. How many grams of NaCl are in 1 L of normal saline?
   Normal saline is 0.9% sodium chloride (NaCl), so there are 0.9 gm of NaCl in 100 ml of normal saline.

$$\frac{0.9 \text{ gm}}{100 \text{ ml}} = \frac{x \text{ gm}}{1000 \text{ ml}} \rightarrow 100x = 0.9 \times 1000 \rightarrow x = \frac{900}{100} \rightarrow x = 9 \text{ gm}$$

example 5.13

If there are 8 g of active ingredient in 240 g of an ointment, what is the W/W%?

$$\frac{8 \text{ g}}{240} = \frac{x \text{ g}}{100}$$

Solve for x by cross-multiplying:

$$240(x) = 8(100)$$

Divide both sides by 240:

$$\frac{240x}{240} = \frac{800}{240}$$

$$x = 3.33$$

Answer: There are 3.33 g of active ingredient in every 100 g of ointment. Therefore, by definition, the percent strength is 3.3%.

example 5.14

If there are 10 g of active ingredient in 500 ml of sodium chloride, what is the W/V%?

$$\frac{10\,g}{500\,ml} = \frac{x\,g}{100\,ml}$$

Solve for x by cross-multiplying:

$$500(x) = 10(100)$$

Divide both sides by 500:

$$\frac{500x}{500} = \frac{1000}{500}$$

$$x = 2$$

Answer: There are 2 g of active ingredient in every 100 ml of sodium chloride. Therefore, by definition, the percent strength of the solution is 2%.

example 5.15

If 40 mL of active ingredient is diluted to 1 L, what is the V/V%?

$$\frac{40\,mL}{1000\,mL} = \frac{x\,mL}{100\,mL}$$

Solve for x by cross-multiplying:

$$1000(x) = 40(100)$$

Divide both sides by 1000:

$$\frac{1000x}{1000} = \frac{4000}{1000}$$

$$x = 4$$

Answer: There are 4 mL of active ingredient in every 100 mL of solution. Therefore, by definition, the percent strength is 4%.

example 5.16

If 1 pint of a solution contains 50 gm of active ingredient, what is the percent strength (W/V)?

$$\frac{50\,gm}{473\,ml} = \frac{x\,gm}{100\,ml}$$

Solve for x by cross-multiplying:

$$473(x) = 50(100)$$

Divide both sides by 473:

$$\frac{473}{473} = \frac{5000}{473}$$

$$x = 10.57$$

Answer: There are 10.57 g of active ingredient in every 100 ml of solution. Therefore, by definition, the percent strength is 10.57%.

example 5.17

If you mix 30 gm of 65% hydrocortisone (HC) with 60 gm of 13% HC, what is the percent strength (W/W) of the final product?

First, we need to determine how many grams of HC are in each individual component.

65% HC:

$$\frac{65\,gm}{100\,gm} = \frac{x\,gm}{30\,gm}$$

Solve for x by cross-multiplying:

$$100(x) = 65(30)$$

Divide both sides by 100:

$$\frac{100x}{100} = \frac{1950}{100}$$

$$x = 19.5$$

Answer: There are 19.5 gm of HC in 30 gm of 65% hydrocortisone.

13%:

$$\frac{13\,gm}{100\,gm} = \frac{x\,gm}{60\,gm}$$

Solve for x by cross-multiplying:

$$100(x) = 60(13)$$

Divide both sides by 100:

$$\frac{100x}{100} = \frac{780}{100}$$

$$x = 7.8$$

Answer: There are 7.8 gm of HC in 60 gm of 13% hydrocortisone.

Therefore, if we mix 30 gm of 65% HC and 60 gm of 13% HC, we will have 90 gm of product containing 27.3 gm of hydrocortisone (19.5 + 7.8).

To determine the final concentration:

$$\frac{x\,gm}{100\,gm} = \frac{27.3\,gm}{90\,gm}$$

Solve for x by cross-multiplying:

$$90(x) = 27.3(100)$$

Divide both sides by 90:

$$\frac{90x}{90} = \frac{2730}{90}$$

$$x = 30.3$$

Answer: $x = 30.3$, so the final concentration of the 90 gm is 30.3%.

Dilutions

Oftentimes a pharmacy has to dilute a concentrated stock solution with distilled or sterile water to compound a less concentrated solution for a prescription. Pharmacies may also dilute a concentrated solid preparation (cream, unguent, paste, etc.) with an inactive ingredient (Aquaphor, Vaseline, lanolin, etc.) to prepare a less concentrated solid preparation. The following formulas can be used for diluting stock solutions or preparations:

initial volume × initial strength = final volume × final strength

$$V_1 \times S_1 = V_2 \times S_2$$

initial quantity × initial strength = final quantity × final strength

$$Q_1 \times S_1 = Q_2 \times S_2$$

initial volume (V_1) or quantity (Q_1) = volume/weight of solution #1 (stock solution)

initial strength (S_1) = strength of solution #1 (stock solution)

final volume (V_2) or quantity (Q_2) = volume/weight of solution #2 (desired solution)

final strength (S_2) = strength of solution #2 (desired solution)

EXAMPLES:

1. How many milliliters of 70% alcohol can be made from 1 pint of 91% alcohol?

$$V_1 \times S_1 = V_2 \times S_2$$

$$473 \text{ ml} \times 91\% = x \text{ ml} \times 70\% \rightarrow 43{,}043 = 70x \rightarrow \frac{43{,}043}{70} = x \rightarrow x = 614.9 \text{ ml}$$

2. How much water will be needed for the previous problem?

total volume prepared (70%) = 614.9 ml

volume of stock solution used (91%) = -473 ml

volume of distilled water needed = 141.9 ml

Therefore, if you dilute 1 pint of 91% alcohol with 141.9 ml of distilled water, you will obtain 614.9 ml of 70% alcohol solution.

3. How many grams of 2.5% hydrocortisone (HC) cream should be mixed with an ointment base to prepare 500 gms of 1% HC?

$$Q_1 \times S_1 = Q_2 \times S_2$$

$$x \text{ gm} \times 2.5\% = 500 \text{ ml} \times 1\% \rightarrow 2.5x = 500 \rightarrow x = \frac{500}{2.5} \rightarrow x = 200 \text{ gm}$$

4. How much of the ointment base will be needed for the previous problem?

total amount prepared (1%) = 500 gm

amount of stock preparation used (2.5%) = -200 gm

volume of distilled water needed = 300 gm

Therefore, you will need to mix 200 gm of 2.5% HC with 300 gm of ointment base to prepare 500 gm of 1% HC.

IMPORTANT

When diluting concentrated stock solutions or preparations, the volume or weight and the strength have to be in the same unit of measure on each side of the equals sign.

EXAMPLE: You need to prepare 473 ml of a 200-mg/ml sorbitol solution. You have only a 70% sorbitol solution available.

Notice that the strengths of the desired solution and the stock solution are not in the same units. The strengths have to be converted to the same unit of measure before they can be plugged into the formula. You can either change 200 mg/ml to percent *or* change 70% to mg/ml.

example 5.18

How much 25% HCl stock solution is required to make 1 oz of 10% HCl solution?

Use the formula $V_1 \times S_1 = V_2 \times S_2$.

$$x \times 25 = 30 \times 10$$
$$25x = 300$$

Divide both sides by 25:

$$\frac{25x}{25} = \frac{300}{25}$$
$$x = 12$$

Answer: Therefore, 12 mL of the 25% stock solution is needed to make 30 mL of the desired solution

Milliequivalents

Milliequivalents (mEq) is a unit of measure that is commonly used in compounding total parenteral nutrition (TPN). These units may look intimidating, but you can treat them like any other unit of measure and make calculations using ratios and proportions.

example 5.19

Electrolyte	Stock Vial	Rx Order	How Many mL?
NaCl	4 mEq/mL	40 mEq	_____

Using the information provided, set up the ratios and proportion to solve:

$$\frac{4\,mEq}{1\,ml} = \frac{40\,mEq}{x\,ml}$$

Cross-multiply:

$$40 = 4x$$

Divide both sides by 4:

$$x = 10$$

So 10 mL of 4-mEq/ml NaCL should be added to the TPN.

Intravenous Flow Rates

IV flow rates are commonly expressed in either ml/hr or gtt/min. When the rate is expressed in ml/hr it is called the IV rate, which is the speed at which an IV solution is infused into a patient. When the rate is expressed in gtt/min it is called the drip rate, which is the speed the IV administration set is calibrated to in order to achieve the IV rate. For example, if a patient has an IV ordered at 100 ml/hr, the nurse has to calculate the drip rate so he can calibrate the IV administration set appropriately to set an IV rate of 100 ml/hr.

FORMULA

IV Rate

$$\frac{\text{volume to be infused (ml)}}{\text{infusion time (hr)}} = \text{ml/hr}$$

EXAMPLE: Rx: D5W 1 L q6h. What is the IV rate?

$$\frac{1000 \text{ ml}}{6} = 166.67 = 167 \text{ ml/hr}$$

IMPORTANT

IV rates should always be rounded to the nearest whole number (ml), because decimals cannot be input into the IV administration pump.

IV Frequency or Schedule

The frequency or schedule of an IV is the time it takes to infuse a specific volume of solution. An IV's frequency/schedule is usually expressed in hours. Do not follow standard rounding rules. Always round an IV's frequency/schedule down to the nearest whole number in hours, as this will ensure that the patient gets enough IV solution.

FORMULA

IV Frequency or Schedule

$$\frac{\text{total volume to be infused}}{\text{IV rate}} = \text{q\_\_\_\_hr}$$

EXAMPLE: Rx: NS 1 L to be infused @ 145 ml/hr. What is the frequency of a 1-L IV bag?

$$\frac{2000 \text{ mL}}{145 \text{ ml/hr}} = 13.79 = \text{q 13 hr}$$

IV Drip Rates

An IV drip rate is used by the caregiver to calibrate the IV administration set to ensure the correct infusion of IV solution. Each IV administration set is labeled with a drop factor (gtt/ml). The drop factor determines how many drops per milliliter are delivered in that particular IV set. Not all IV sets have the same drop factor. Be sure you know the correct drop factor before beginning.

FORMULA

IV Drip Rate

$$\frac{\text{volume to be infused (ml)}}{\text{infusion time (min)}} \times \text{IV set drop factor} = \text{drops/min}$$

---

example 5.20

Rx: D5W, 400 mL to run over 4 hr. IV drop factor: 10 gtt/mL. Determine the rate of infusion in gtt/min.

$$\frac{400\,\text{mL}}{240\,\text{min}} \times \frac{10\,\text{gtt}}{\text{ml}} = \text{gtt/min}$$

Cancel like units before solving:

$$\frac{400\,\cancel{\text{mL}}}{240\,\text{min}} \times \frac{10\,\text{gtt}}{\cancel{\text{ml}}} = \text{gtt/min}$$

Multiply across (400 × 10) and divide by 240 to get the answer.

Answer: 16.67 ≈ 17 gtt/min.

---

example 5.21

Rx: NS 2 L IV q24h. IV drop factor: 60 gtt/mL.

$$\frac{2000\,\text{mL}}{1440\,\text{min}} \times \frac{60\,\text{gtt}}{\text{ml}} = \text{gtt/min}$$

Cancel like units before solving:

$$\frac{2000\,\cancel{\text{mL}}}{1440\,\text{min}} \times \frac{60\,\text{gtt}}{\cancel{\text{ml}}} = \text{gtt/min}$$

Multiply across (2000 × 60) and divide by 1440 to get the answer.

Answer: 83.33 ≈ 83 gtt/min.

Alligations

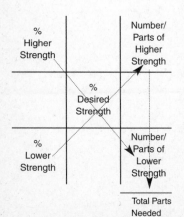

Alligations are used when mixing together two different strengths of the same active ingredient, so that the strength of the final product is the one that is desired. You can solve alligation problems easily by using the alligation grid shown below. First, input the amount of the higher strength, the lower strength, and the desired strength. Then take the difference on the diagonals (which should always be a positive number) to determine the number or part needed. To finish solving the alligation, read across the grid as you would a book, from left to right. The number or parts of the higher strength needed should be listed as a fraction of the total number of parts needed—which is solved by simply adding the numbers in the right column.

If you are using a solvent or diluent such as water, cream/ointment base, or normal saline (assuming that sodium chloride is not the active ingredient), use a percent strength of zero since it contains no active ingredient.

example 5.22

Rx: Hydrocortisone 5% cream, 120 gm. You have in stock 2% hydrocortisone cream and 10% hydrocortisone cream. How much of each should be used to make 120 g of 5% hydrocortisone cream?

Set up an alligation grid:

% Higher Strength 10		Number/ Parts of Higher Strength 3
	% Desired Strength 5	
% Lower Strength 2		Number/ Parts of Lower Strength 5
		Total Parts Needed: 8

To make this order you should use 3 parts (out of 8 total parts) of the 10% cream and 5 parts (out of 8 total parts) of the 2% cream. Because we know the proportion required and the total amount needed, we can calculate the actual amount required of each product by multiplying the total quantity by the proportion needed:

$$\text{quantity of 10\% HC needed: } 120\,\text{g} \times 3/8 = 45\,\text{g}$$
$$\text{quantity of 2\% HC needed: } 120\,\text{g} \times 5/8 = 75\,\text{g}$$

Therefore, if you mix 45 g of 10% HC cream with 75 g of 2% HC cream, the resulting 120 g of HC cream will have a strength of 5%.

example 5.23

Rx: Clotrimazole 0.5% ointment. How much 10% clotrimazole powder and ointment base should be mixed together to prepare 240 g of ointment?

Set up an alligation grid:

10%		0.5
	0.5%	
0% (ointment base contains no active ingredient)		9.5
		Total Parts Needed: 10

To make this order you should use 0.5 parts (out of 10 total parts) of the 10% and 9.5 parts (out of 10 total parts) of the ointment base cream. Because we know the proportion required and the total amount needed, we can calculate the actual amount required of each product by multiplying the total quantity by the proportion needed:

$$\text{quantity of 10\% clotrimazole needed: } 240\,\text{g} \times 0.5/10 = 12\,\text{g}$$
$$\text{quantity of 2\% clotrimazole needed: } 240\,\text{g} \times 9.5/10 = 228\,\text{g}$$

Therefore, if you mix 12 g of 10% clotrimazole powder with 228 g of ointment base, the resulting 240 g of clotrimazole cream will be at a strength of 0.5%.

Business Math

Although pharmacy technicians do not have to be accountants, they must have a basic understanding of the accounting and business calculations that are used in many practice settings. Following are the most common business math calculation formulas used in pharmacy.

FORMULA

Selling Price, Cost, and Markup

$$\text{Selling price} = \text{Cost} + \text{Markup}$$

FORMULA

Calculating Markup Percentage

$$\text{Markup percentage} = \frac{(\text{Selling price} - \text{Cost})}{\text{Cost}} \times 100$$

FORMULA

Calculating Gross Profit

$$\text{Selling price} - \text{Invoice cost} = \text{Gross profit}$$

FORMULA

Calculating Gross Profit Percentage

$$\frac{(\text{Price} - \text{Cost})}{\text{Cost}} \times 100 = \text{Gross profit percentage}$$

FORMULA

Calculating Net Profit

$$\text{Net profit} = \text{Selling price} - (\text{Cost} + \text{Overhead})$$

example 5.24

A blood pressure monitor costs the pharmacy $18.65, and the store adds a 20% markup to all medical devices. What is the selling price of the monitor?

$$\text{Selling price} = \$18.65 + (\$18.65 \times 20\%)$$
$$= \$18.65 + \$3.73$$
$$= \$22.38$$

example 5.25

A bottle of 81-mg aspirin is priced at $2.89; the invoice cost is $1.98. What is the amount of the markup, and what is the markup percentage?

$$\$2.89 = \$1.98 + \text{markup}$$

Subtract $1.98 from both sides:

$$\$0.82 = \text{markup}$$

To determine the markup percentage, use the other formula:

$$\begin{aligned} \text{Markup \%} &= (\$2.89 - \$1.98)/\$1.98 \times 100 \\ &= \$0.82/\$1.98 \times 100 \\ &= 41.4\% \end{aligned}$$

Practice Problems

To Practice the calculations from this chapter, please take the Math Practice Tests in chapters 13, 14, and 15.

SUMMARY

Many pharmacy technicians find pharmacy calculations to be the most difficult aspect of pharmacy practice; however, a very large part of pharmacy practice and of the national certification exam focuses on calculations. It is important to remember that no matter how intimidating these pharmacy calculations may seem at first glance, most can be solved either by using simple ratios and proportions or by using an algebraic formula. It is important for pharmacy technicians to master these calculations, not only for the national exam but to function successfully on the job and, most important, for patient safety.

CHAPTER REVIEW QUESTIONS

1. Rx: Albuterol 2 mg/5 mL, 1.5 tsp po bid. Disp: 120 ml. How many milligrams of albuterol will be taken per day?

   a. 6 mg   c. 10 mg
   b. 12 mg   d. 20 mg

2. Rx: Amoxicillin/potassium clavulante, 45 mg/kg/day in 3 divided doses. The patient weighs 54 lb. How many milligrams will the patient receive for each dose?

   a. 2430 mg
   b. 368.25 mg
   c. 810 mg
   d. 1105 mg

3. 480 ml = _____ tsp

   a. 32   c. 64
   b. 48   d. 96

4. 3.5 gallons = _____ ml

   a. 3785   c. 13,320
   b. 14,000   d. 13,249

5. Rx: D5 ½ NS 1 L IV q8h. What is the IV rate?

   a. 80 ml/hr
   b. 120 ml/hr
   c. 125 ml/hr
   d. 75 ml/hr
   e. 90 ml/hr

6. Rx: ½ NS IV @ 75 ml/hr. What is the frequency of a 1-L IV bag?

   a. q12h
   b. q13h
   c. q14h
   d. q24h

7.

Electrolyte	Stock Vial	Rx Order	How Many mL?
KCl	2 mEq/mL	90 mEq	_____

   a. 60 mL
   b. 15 mL
   c. 10 mL
   d. 30 mL
   e. 45 mL

8. How many milliliters of 2.7% NaCl need to be added to distilled water to make 1 L of normal saline?

   a. 333 mL
   b. 667 mL
   c. 500 mL
   d. 250 mL

9. Rx: PenVK 500,000 units in 50 mL is to be administered over 30 minutes. The IV set drop factor of 20 gtt/ml. What is the infusion rate in drops per minute?

   a. 1.6 gtt/min
   b. 3.3 gtt/min
   c. 16 gtt/min
   d. 33 gtt/min
   e. 333 gtt/min

10. What is the markup percentage on a box of latex gloves that is invoiced at $3.39 and sold for $5.36?

   a. 42%
   b. 73%
   c. 58%
   d. 27%

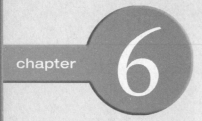

6 Pharmacy Law and Ethics

After completing this chapter, you should be able to:

- Describe pharmacy laws that affect everyday pharmacy practice.
- Explain the intent of pharmacy laws.
- Describe major pieces of federal pharmacy legislation and explain how they affect the practice of pharmacy.
- State the intent of the Poison Prevention Packaging Act (PPPA) and list exceptions to it.
- Define theories of ethical reasoning.
- Explain the importance of law and ethics in pharmacy practice.
- Compare the differences between lawful and ethical behavior.

Introduction

The pharmacy laws in the United States are complicated and multifaceted. Although laws are ultimately created to preserve peace, order, and public safety, in a free society, politics, finance, power, and influence can also play role. Pharmacy laws, rules, regulations, and ethical standards have been developed over the years to increase public safety by protecting consumers, regulating the pharmacy profession, and requiring acccountability of the pharmaceutical industry.

Pharmacy laws are not new; they date back to the thirteenth century, when Holy Roman Emperor Frederick II decreed a separation of the practice of medicine and the study of drugs, thus creating the pharmacy profession. After promulgation of this decree, doctors studied disease states and the human body, and apothecaries (pharmacists) studied how drugs worked and their effects on the human body.

Unfortunately, as with most laws, sometimes something has to go terribly wrong before a new pharmacy law is enacted. It is usually not until a group of people say, "There ought to be a law!" or someone is injured or dies that many laws are passed. Pharmacy laws are also passed because of a loophole or oversight in a previous law.

Because each state has its own specific pharmacy laws, rules, and regulations that govern the practice of pharmacy in that state, national pharmacy technician exams only ask questions regarding federal law. Therefore, this chapter focuses on major pieces of federal pharmacy legislation that have affected today's practice of pharmacy.

Food and Drug Act of 1906

By the end of the nineteenth century, opium, morphine, and cocaine were commonly used and were available almost everywhere, including in grocery stores. Consumers were becoming addicted to miracle cures touted as secret elixirs and cure-alls containing what we now consider dangerous substances.

The purpose of this law the Food and Drug Act of 1906 was to prohibit interstate commerce of misbranded or adulterated food and drugs in the United States. False claims used to advertise the drug failed to hold up in court as "misbranding." Additionally, the act did not grant any legal authority to any government agency to ban or recall any drugs that might protentially be unsafe. Rather than put a false label on a drug, the manufacturer could just leave off the label and not list ingredients at all. Six years later, in 1912, Congress passed an amendment that included in the definition of misbranding any false or fraudulent claims of the curative powers of drugs.

International Opium Convention of 1912

Narcotic abuse and addiction was not confined to the United States: The problem was worldwide. At a convention at The Hague in 1912, many nations signed the first international agreement creating controlled substances.

The purpose of the agreement was to limit the import and export of opium to licensed individuals only; prevent all opium prepared for smoking from import or export; begin the first tracking of controlled substances from manufacture to import, export, and distribution; and limit the use of these substances to medical cases. Although the United States signed the international agreement, it had no laws in effect to ensure compliance by citizens.

Narcotic Drug Act of 1914

The Narcotic Drug Act of 1914, also known as the Harrison Narcotic Act, states that "every person who produces, imports, manufactures, compounds, deals in, dispenses, distributes, or gives away opium or coca leaves or any compound, manufacture, salt, derivative, or preparation thereof, shall register" and pay appropriate taxes. Now physicians, pharmacists, importers, and manufacturers had to be licensed to prescribe narcotics. The law did not affect the dispensing of narcotics during the "course of professional practice." This clause, however, was ambiguous, and many physicians were arrested, convicted, and imprisoned for prescribing opitate to addicts, because addiction was not considered a disease and therefore did not fall under "professional practice."

Food, Drug, and Cosmetic Act of 1938

In 1937, sulfa-based drugs were considered the "miracle drugs" of their time and were commonly dispensed in powder form. However, manufacturers reasoned that even small children could benefit by taking it in liquid form as a remedy for sore throats. The problem was getting the powder to dissolve. The only medium that seemed to work was diethylene glycol. More than 100 children died after taking sulfanilamide that was dissolved in diethylene glycol. Today, we know that diethylene glycol is a deadly poison used commonly in automobile radiators.

The furor over the sulfanilamide disaster prompted a cry for greater public safety, and the idea that a drug could be marketed without manufacturer assurance that it would not kill suddenly became unacceptable. Up to that time, there was no guarantee that any medication was safe for human consumption.

The purpose of the Food, Drug, and Cosmetic Act was to require adequate testing of drugs to ensure their safety for human consumption. This law defines *safe* as "nontoxic when used in accordance with the conditions set forth on the label." The law created the Food and Drug Adminsitration (FDA) and now required new drugs to go testing before being placed on the market. Drugs available before this time, such as phenobarbital and digoxin, were "grandfathered" and not subject to the new legislation.

Although drugs were now being tested for safety, the law did not require drugs to be effective. It was not until 1949 that batch certification was required for antibiotics to assure their potency and efficacy. The law also included the following requirements for retail prescription labels: name and address of pharmacy, prescription number, date filled, name of patient, directions for use, and cautionary statements.

Durham-Humphrey Amendment of 1951

The Durham-Humphrey Amendment was the first law to distinguish between over-the-counter (OTC) drugs and prescription or legend drugs, in that prescription drugs now had to bear the legend, "Caution: Federal Law Prohibits Dispensing Without a Prescription." Later amendments approved a substitute legend that simply reads "Rx only." The act also allowed for verbal prescriptions and refills.

Kefauver-Harris Amendment of 1962

In the late 1950s and early 1960s, a drug called thalidomide was commonly prescribed as a sleep aid, especially in Europe, where it was also often taken by pregnant women to control morning sickness. Unfortunately, it was discovered that women who took thalidomide in their first trimester of pregnancy often gave birth to babies with birth defects (primarily missing or very small limbs). The situation became even worse as some women decided on abortions, which were illegal at the time. It became clear that doctors, prescribers, and drug manufacturers often did not have a clear picture of a drug's reactions or interactions, and that prescribers and patients were relying on information supplied by the manufacturer, which was not complete and sometimes was deliberately falsified or suppressed.

In 1962, the Kefauver-Harris Amendment was passed in an attempt to identify and define drug efficacy. The purpose of the admendment was to hold manufacturers accountable for their drug products and to require inspection of manufacturing sites. Manufacturers now had to:

- Supply proof of effectiveness
- Supply proof of safety
- Follow Good Manufacturing Practices (GMPs) set by the government
- Answer to the Food and Drug Administration (FDA) for advertising practices and claims

- Follow specific procedures requiring informed consent waivers and reporting of adverse drug reactions while a drug was being developed

Poison Prevention Packaging Act of 1970

The Poison Prevention Packaging Act (PPPA) authorized the Consumer Product Safety Commission (CPSC) to create standards for child-resistant packaging, requiring OTC and legend drugs (unless exempt) to be packaged in child-resistant containers. A child-resistant container is one that cannot be opened by 80% of children under the age of five years but that can be opened by 90% of adults. The prescriber or adult patient can request a "non–child-resistant" container. However, the pharmacy must include the information on the patient's record and usually requires a signed release form.

Exemptions to the PPPA requirements include drugs dispensed by institutional pharmacies and administered by institutional employees, inhalation aerosols, oral contraceptives, sublingual nitroglycerin, sublingual and chewable isosorbide dinitrate (10 mg or less), methylprednisolone tablets (<85 mg per package), and prednisone tablets (<105 mg per package). Visit www.cpsc.gov for a complete listing of exempt drugs.

Comprehensive Drug Abuse Prevention and Control Act of 1970

The purpose of the Comprehensive Drug Abuse Prevention and Control Act was to consolidate all existing federal laws dealing with narcotic drugs, stimulants, depressants, and other drugs with abuse potential and required the pharmaceutical industry to keep strict records and ensure the physical security of these drugs.

This act, commonly called the Controlled Substance Act (CSA), classified controlled substances into one of five categories based on their abuse potential. The CSA also led to the consolidation of several federal governmental agencies by creating the Drug Enforcement Administration to enforce the new laws and to fight drug abuse and diversion.

Orphan Drug Act of 1983

Orphan drugs are drugs that are used to treat rare diseases that affect less than 1 out of 200,000 people. The Orphan Drug Act offers financial and licensing incentives to manufacturers to research and develop drugs for these rare diseases. Currently there are over 300 orphan drugs.

Omnibus Budget Reconciliation Act of 1990

The Omnibus Budget Reconciliation Act of 1990 (OBRA) now required pharmacists to provide prospective drug use review (ProDUR), conduct patient counseling, and maintain proper patient records in order to receive reimbursment for Medicaid prescriptions. Pharmacists are now busy consulting and counseling, so technicians have become even more important to the operation of a pharmacy: Good technicians need to know more and do more. It is important for technicians to recognize the value of pharmacist counseling and to support that service by freeing the pharmacist's time. In most states, the three requirements of OBRA are now required for all patients, not just Medicaid patients.

Americans with Disabilities Act of 1990

The Americans with Disabilities Act (ADA) is a federal law that prohibits discrimination based on any disability. The act states that "no covered entity shall discriminate against a qualified individual on the basis of disability in regard to job application procedures, the hiring, advancement, or discharge of employees, employee compensation, job training, and other terms, conditions, and privileges of employment." For more information, visit www.ada.gov.

Health Insurance Portability and Accountability Act of 1996

Provisions of the Health Insurance Portability and Accountability Act of 1996 (HIPAA) that affect pharmacy practice include:

- **Standards for electronic health information transactions.** This includes standards for electronic health care–related transactions such as claims and payments as well as security for health information systems.
- **Privacy.** This provision requires that all patient personal and health-related information be protected and remain private. It sets guidelines that require patients to be informed about how their personal information is shared and/or used. It requires that all patient information be kept confidential and be used only as needed. Pharmacy technicians cannot, under any circumstances, release protected information to any unauthorized individual.
- **Penalties.** Providers and health plans (including pharmacy technicians) are subject to civil penalties and prison terms for violations.

HIPAA also requires all employees who handle health-related information to be trained and reviewed annually. Violations of company HIPAA rules by a pharmacy technician could result in immediate termination of employment. For more information visit www.hhs.gov/ocr/hipaa.

Medicare Prescription Drug, Improvement, and Modernization Act of 2003

The Medicare Prescription Drug, Improvement, and Modernization Act (MMA) is also known as Medicare Part D and allows patients with Medicare health insurance to add prescription drug coverage, which may lower their prescription drug costs and help protect against higher costs in the future. Medicare prescription drug coverage is insurance that is provided by private companies. Participants choose a drug plan, and most pay a monthly premium. Beneficiaries who do not enroll in a drug plan when they first become eligible may be subject to a penalty if they choose to enroll later. For more information, visit www.cms.hhs.gov.

Combat Methamphetamine Epidemic Act of 2006

The Combat Methamphetamine Epidemic Act (CMEA) regulates retail over-the-counter sales of ephedrine, pseudoephedrine, and phenylpropanolamine products, all which are precursor chemicals used in the illegal manufacture of methamphetamines or amphetamines. Retail provisions of the CMEA include daily sales limits of 3.6 g and monthly purchase limits of 9 g by each purchaser. The products must be placed out of direct customer access, either behind the pharmacy counter or under lock and key. Pharmacies are also required to keep sales logbooks, verify customer IDs, and conduct employee training.

Ethics

The practice of pharmacy is one of the most heavily regulated industries of our time. How, then, do professional pharmacy technicians reconcile their actions with their own moral, ethical, and legal standards? The law is the law, but is it right? More important, is it ethical?

Ethics can be defined as the rules or standards governing the conduct of a person or the members of a profession, the science of human nature or system of principles governing morally correct conduct. Ethics are more than law; they are used to guide professionals in making decisions when the "correct" course of action may be unclear or uncertain. Technicians can think of ethics as the accepted standards of conduct for the pharmacy profession.

At the same time, pharmacy technicians must realize that not every situation they may encounter will have a rule or regulation that dictates their proper response or behavior. For example, pharmacy law does not usually mandate that a pharmacy choose the best-priced medication for a patient, but pharmacy ethics do. One must also remember that a profession's ethical standards may not necessarily be aligned with one's own personal moral and religious beliefs.

Each technician has many decisions to make every day. These decisions profoundly affect the people we serve, the people we work with, and the pharmacists we assist. Our decisions and actions must be well thought out, carefully considered, and not just knee-jerk, emotional, or blindly legal behaviors.

Code of Ethics

To aid pharmacy technicians in their decision-making and professional behavior, the American Association of Pharmacy Technicians (AAPT) has adopted the following pharmacy technician code of ethics.

Preamble

Pharmacy technicians are healthcare professional who assist pharmacists in providing the best possible care for patients. The principles of this code, which apply to pharmacy technicians working in any and all settings, are based on the application and support of the moral obligations that guide the pharmacy profession in relationships with patients, healthcare professionals and society.

Principles

I. A pharmacy technician's first consideration is to ensure the health and safety of the patient and to use knowledge and skills to the best of his/her ability in serving others.

II. A pharmacy technician supports and promotes honesty and integrity in the profession, which includes a duty to observe the law, maintain the highest moral and ethical conduct at all times and uphold the ethical principles of the profession.

III. A pharmacy technician assists and supports the pharmacist in the safe, efficacious and cost-effective distribution of health services and health care resources.

IV. A pharmacy technician respects and values the abilities of pharmacists, colleagues, and other healthcare professionals.

V. A pharmacy technician maintains competency in his/her practice and continually enhances his/her professional knowledge and expertise.

VI. A pharmacy technician respects and supports the patient's individuality, dignity, and confidentiality.

VII. A pharmacy technician respects the confidentiality of a patient's records and discloses pertinent information only with proper authorization.

VIII. A pharmacy technician never assists in the dispensing, promoting, or distributing of medications or medical devices that are not of good quality or do not meet the standards required by law.

IX. A pharmacy technician does not engage in any activity that will discredit the profession and will expose, without fear or favor, illegal, or unethical conduct in the profession.

X. A pharmacy technician associates with and engages in the support of organizations which promote the profession of pharmacy through the use and enhancement of pharmacy technicians.

SUMMARY

The topic of law and ethics in pharmacy is diverse, complex, and comprehensive. The practice of pharmacy is regulated by both federal and state agencies, but it is impossible to list the specifics of law in each state. Moreover, the national exam focuses only on federal law, not state laws. Therefore, this chapter has reviewed the federal laws and ethical principles that are covered by the national certification exam.

CHAPTER REVIEW QUESTIONS

1. Which law made the initial distinction between OTC and legend drugs?
   a. Pure Food and Drug Act
   b. Food, Drug, and Cosmetic Act
   c. Durham-Humphrey Amendment
   d. Kefauver-Harris Amendment

2. Which law restricted the interstate commerce of misbranded or adulterated drugs?
   a. Pure Food and Drug Act
   b. Food, Drug, and Cosmetic Act
   c. Durham-Humphrey Amendment
   d. Kefauver-Harris Amendment

3. Which law was enacted in an effort to make sure that drugs are safe for human consumption?
   a. Pure Food and Drug Act
   b. Food, Drug, and Cosmetic Act
   c. Durham-Humphrey Amendment
   d. Kefauver-Harris Amendment

4. Which law requires technicians to maintain patient confidentiality?
   a. OBRA
   b. Food, Drug, and Cosmetic Act
   c. Durham-Humphrey Amendment
   d. HIPAA

5. Which law requires drugs to be both safe and effective for their labeled use?
   a. OBRA
   b. Food, Drug, and Cosmetic Act

   c. Durham-Humphrey Amendment
   d. Kefauver-Harris Amendment
   e. HIPAA

6. _____ required pharmacists to provide patient counseling to _____ patients.
   a. OBRA, Medicare
   b. HIPAA, Medicaid
   c. OBRA, Medicaid
   d. HIPAA, Medicare

7. Ethics are written guidelines for professional behavior mandated by state boards of pharmacy.
   a. true
   b. false

8. The pharmacy technician code of ethics was established by:
   a. state boards of pharmacy
   b. NPTA
   c. ASHP
   d. AAPT
   e. FDA

9. Which law was passed in response to sulfanilimide deaths?
   a. OBRA
   b. Food, Drug, and Cosmetic Act
   c. Durham-Humphrey Amendment
   d. Kefauver-Harris Amendment
   e. HIPAA

10. Which of the following is *not* a principle of the pharmacy technician code of ethics?

    a. A pharmacy technician's first consideration is to ensure the health and safety of the patient and to use knowledge and skills to the best of his/her ability in serving others.

    b. A pharmacy technician should always fill and deliver patient prescriptions within 15 minutes.

    c. A pharmacy technician is honest in professional business dealings including those with clients, third party payers and suppliers of drugs, non-prescription medications and health related products.

    d. A pharmacy technician respects the confidentiality of a patient's records and discloses pertinent information only with proper authorization.

7 Top 200 Drugs

Introduction

Listed in the following table are the top 200 most commonly dispensed medications in the United States. Although the top 200 list changes every year, many drugs remain on the list for many years. Pharmacy technicians should be familiar with these medications so they can assist both pharmacists and patients. As a working technician as well as to pass the national certification exam, it is a major responsibility to recognize brand and generic names; know dosage forms, classifications, and strengths; and to know which auxiliary labels should be used with which drug. Making your own personal set of flash cards using index cards is a great way to quiz yourself and to prepare for the national exam.

When choosing a drug product, it is important for pharmacy technicians to pay close attention to the name of the drug, because many drugs are similar in spelling and sound, which makes it easy to mistake one drug for another. Thereore, also included in this chapter is the Joint Commission's list of look-alike, sound-alike drugs.

If the drug is a controlled substance, the schedule is listed after the generic name.

GENERIC NAME	BRAND NAME	CLASS	STRENGTH/DOSAGE FORM
Acetaminophen with codeine (CIII)	Tylenol, Phenaphen (with codeine)	Narcotic analgesic	#3 tab = 300 mg acetaminophen, 30 mg codeine #4 tab = 300 mg acetaminophen, 60 mg codeine
Acyclovir	Zovirax	Antiviral	200-mg cap 400-mg, 800-mg tab 200-mg/5-ml susp 50-mg/ml inj 5% cream and oint
Albuterol sulfate (inhalation)	Proventil, Ventolin, Proair	Beta$_2$ agonist (antiasthmatic)	2-mg, 4-mg tab 4-mg, 8-mg ER tab 200-mcg cap for inhalation 0.083%, 0.5% inhalation soln 90-mcg/acuation inhalation aerosol
Alendronate sodium	Fosamax	Osteoporosis agent (bisphosphonate derivative)	5-mg, 10-mg, 35-mg, 40-mg, 70-mg tab 70-mg/75-ml oral soln
Allopurinol	Zyloprim	Anti-gout agent	100-mg, 300-mg tab 500=mg inj
Alprazolam (CIV)	Xanax, Xanax XR	Antianxiety agent (BZD)	0.25-mg, 0.5-mg, 1-mg, 2-mg tab 0.5-mg, 1-mg, 2-mg, 3-mg SR tab 0.5-mg/5-ml, 1-mg/ml oral soln 0.25-mg, 0.5-mg, 1-mg, 2-mg disintegrating tab
Amiodarone	Cordarone, Pacerone	Antiarrhythmic (Class III)	
Amitriptyline HCl	Elavil	Antidepressant (TCA)	10-mg, 25-mg, 50-mg, 75-mg, 100-mg, 150-mg tab 10-mg/ml inj
Amlodipine besylate	Norvasc	Antihypertensive (CCB)	2.5-mg, 5-mg, 10-mg tab
Amlodipine besylate with atorvastatin Ca	Caduet	Antihypertensive/ antilipidemic	2.5-mg/10-mg, 2.5-mg/20-mg, 2.5-mg/40-mg, 5-mg/10-mg, 5-mg/20-mg, 5-mg/40-mg, 5-mg/80-mg, 10-mg/10-mg, 10-mg/20-mg, 10-mg/40-mg, 10-mg/80-mg tab
Amlodipine besylate with benazepril HCl	Lotrel	Antihypertensive (CCB/ACE-I)	2.5-mg/10-mg, 5-mg/10-mg, 5-mg/20-mg, 5-mg/40-mg, 10-mg/20-mg, 10-mg/40-mg tab
Amoxicillin trihydrate	Amoxil, Trimox	Penicillin antibiotic	125-mg, 250-mg, 500-mg tab 250-mg, 500-mg cap 50-mg/ml, 125-mg/5-ml, 250-mg/5-ml susp 200-mg, 400-mg, 600=mg dispersible tab
Amoxicillin with clavulanate potassium	Augmentin, Augmentin XR	Penicillin antibiotic	250-mg, 500-mg, 875-mg tab 125-mg, 200-mg, 400-mg chewable tab 125-mg/5-ml, 200-mg/5-ml, 250-mg/5-ml, 400-mg/5ml, 600-mg/5-ml susp

(Continued)

GENERIC NAME	BRAND NAME	CLASS	STRENGTH/DOSAGE FORM
Amphetamine with dextroamphetamine salts (CII)	Adderall, Adderall XR	ADHD agent (CNS stimulant)	5-mg, 10-mg, 20-mg, 30-mg tab 5-mg, 15-mg, 20-mg, 25-mg, 30-mg SR cap
Anastrozole	Arimidex	Antineoplastic (nonsteroidal aromatase inhibitor)	1-mg tab
Aripiprazole	Abilify	Atypic antipsychotic	10-mg, 15-mg, 20-mg, 30-mg tab 1-mg/ml soln
Aspirin, enteric-coated	(Generic)	Salisilate (blood modifier, cox inhibitor)	81-mg, 165-mg, 325-mg, 500-mg, 650-mg, 975-mg EC tab
Atenelol with chlorthalidone	Tenoretic	Antihypertensive	
Atenolol	Tenormin	Antihypertensive (beta blocker)	25-mg, 50-mg, 100-mg tab 5-mg/10-ml vial
Atomoxetine HCl	Strattera	Selective NE reuptake inhibitor (ADHD agent)	10-mg, 18-mg, 25-mg, 40-mg, 60-mg cap
Atorvastatin calcium	Lipitor	Antihyperlipidemic (HMGCoA reductase inhibitor)	10-mg, 20-mg, 40-mg tab
Azelastine HCl (nasal)	Astelin	Antihistamine	137-mcg/spray
Azithromycin dihydrate	Zithromax, Zmax	Macrolide antibiotic	250-mg, 500-mg, 600-mg tab 100-mg/5-ml, 200-mg/5-ml, 1-g/pkt susp 500-mg inj Zmax: 176-mg/5-ml ER susp
Baclofen	Lioresal, Kemstro	Skeletal-muscle relaxant (GABA analog)	10-mg, 20-mg tab 10-mg, 20-mg disintegrating tab 50-mcg/ml, 250-mcg/ml ampoule
Benazepril HCl	Lotensin	Antihypertensive (ACE inhibitor)	5-mg, 10-mg, 20-mg, 40-mg tab
Benazepril with hydrochlorothiazide	Lotensin HCT	Antihypertensive	5-mg/6.25-mg, 10-mg/12.5-mg, 20-mg/12.5-mg, 20-mg/25-mg tab
Benzonatate	Tessalon	Antitussive	100-mg cap
Benztropine mesylate	Cogentin	Anticholinergic (antiparkinson agent)	0.5-mg, 1-mg, 2-mg tab 1-mg/ml ampoule
Bimatoprost	Lumigan	Agent for glaucoma	0.03% ophth soln
Bisoprolol fumarate with HCTZ	Ziac	Antihypertensive	2.5-mg/6.25-mg, 5-mg/6.25-mg, 10-mg/6.25-mg tab
Brimonidine tartrate	Alphagan P	Agent for glaucoma (alpha$_2$ agonist)	0.1%, 0.15% ophth soln
Budenoside (inhalation)	Pulmicort	Corticosteroid (antiasthmatic)	32-mcg/inhalation
Budenoside (nasal)	Rhinocort Aqua	Corticosteroid (antiallergy)	32-mcg nasal spray
Bumetanide	Bumex	Loop diuretic	0.5-mg, 1-mg, 2-mg tab 0.25-mg/ml inj
Bupropion HCl	Wellbutrin, Wellbutrin SR, Wellbutrin XL	Antidepressant	75-mg, 100-mg tab 100-mg, 150-mg, 200-mg SR tab 150-mg, 300-mg ER tab

GENERIC NAME	BRAND NAME	CLASS	STRENGTH/DOSAGE FORM
Buspirone HCl	BuSpar	Non-BZD antianxiety agent	5-mg, 10-mg, 15-mg tab
Butalbital, acetaminophen, and caffeine	Fioricet	Analgesic	50-mg/325-mg/40-mg tab
Candesartan cilexetil	Atacand	Angiotensin receptor blocker (antihypertensive)	4-mg, 8-mg, 16-mg, 32-mg tab
Captopril	Capoten	ACE inhibitor (antihypertensive)	12.5-mg, 25-mg, 50-mg, 100-mg tab
Carbamazepine	Tegretol, Tegretol XR, Carbatrol ER, Equetrol ER	Anticonvulsant	100-mg chewable tab 200-mg tab 100-mg, 200-mg, 400-mg SR tab 100-mg, 200-mg, 300-mg SR cap 100-mg/5-ml susp
Carbidopa with levodopa	Sinemet	Antiparkinson agent (dopaminergic)	10-mg/100-mg, 25-mg/100-mg, 25-mg/250-mg tab 25-mg/100-mg, 50-mg/200-mg SR and disintegrating tab
Carisoprodol	Soma	Skeletal-muscle relaxant	350-mg tab
Carvedilol	Coreg, Coreg CR	Beta blocker (antihypertensive)	3.125-mg, 6.25-mg, 12.5-mg, 25-mg tab
Cefdinir	Omnicef	Cephalosporin antibiotic	300-mg cap 125-mg/5-ml susp
Cefprozil	Cefzil	Cephalosporin antibiotic	250-mg, 500-mg tab 125-mg/5-ml, 250-mg/5-ml susp
Cefuroxime axetil (oral)	Ceftin	Cephalosporin antibiotic	125-mg, 250-mg, 500-mg tab 125-mg/5-ml, 250-mg/5-ml susp
Celecoxib	Celebrex	NSAID (COX2 inhibitor)	100-mg, 200-mg, 400-mg cap
Cephalexin monohydrate	Kelfex	Cephalosporin antibiotic	250-mg, 500-mg cap 250-mg, 500-mg, 1-g tab 125-mg/5-ml, 250-mg/5-ml susp
Cetirizine HCl	Zyrtec	Nonsedating antihistamine (antiallergy)	5-mg, 10-mg tab 5-mg, 10-mg chewable tab 5-mg/5-ml syrup
Chlorhexidine gluconate	Peridex, Periogard	Antiplaque rinse (antimicrobial)	0.12% oral rinse
Hydrocodone polyisterix/ chlorpheniramine polyisterix (CIII)	Tussionex	Antihistamine/ antitussive	10-mg/8-mg per 5 ml
Ciprofloxacin HCl	Cipro, Cipro XR	Fluoroquinolone antibiotic	100-mg, 250-mg, 500-mg 750-mg tab 500-mg ER tab 50-mg/ml, 100-mg/ml susp 200-mg, 400-mg inj 3.5-mg/ml ophth soln
Ciprofloxacin with dexamethasone (otic)	CiproDex	Otic antibiotic/ anti-inflammatory	0.3%/0.1% otic susp

(Continued)

GENERIC NAME	BRAND NAME	CLASS	STRENGTH/DOSAGE FORM
Citalopram HBr	Celexa	SSRI (antidepressant)	20-mg, 40-mg tab 10-mg/5-ml oral soln
Clarithromycin	Biaxin, Biaxin XL	Macrolide antibiotic	250-mg, 500-mg tab 500-mg SR tab 125-mg/5-ml, 250-mg/5-ml susp
Clindamycin HCl (oral)	Cleocin	Antibiotic	75-mg, 150-mg, 300-mg caps 75-mg/5-ml oral susp
Clindamycin phosphate (topical)	Cleocin T	Topical acne treatment	2% vaginal cream 100-mg supp 10-mg gel and lotion 1% foam
Clobetasol propionate (topical)	Temovate	Topical corticosteroid (anti-inflammatory)	0.05% cream
Clonazepam	Klonopin	Benzodiazepine (sedative hypnotic)	0.5-mg, 1-mg, 2-mg tab 0.125-mg, 0.25-mg, 0.5-mg, 1-mg, 2-mg oral disintegrating wafer
Clonidine HCl	Catapress, Catapress TTS	Antihypertensive (central alpha agonist)	0.1-mg, 0.2-mg, 0.3-mg tab 0.1-mg/24-h, 0.2-mg/24-h, 0.3-mg/2-h transdermal patch 100-mcg/ml, 500-mcg/ml inj
Clopidogrel bisulfate	Plavix	Antiplatelet agent	75-mg tab
Clotrimazole with betamethasone dipropionate	Lotrisone	Topical antifungal/ corticosteroid	Topical cream
Codeine phosphate with guaifenesin (CV)	Mytussin AC, Robitussin AC	Antitussive/ expectorant	10-mg/100-mg per 5 ml
Colchicine	Colchicine	Anti-gout agent	0.5-mg, 0.6-mg tab
Cyclobenzaprine HCl	Flexeril, Amrix, Fexmid	Skeletal-muscle relaxant	5-mg, 10-mg tab
Cyclosporine emulsion (ophthalmic)	Restasis	Dry-eye agent/ immunosuppresant	0.05% ophth emulsion
Desloratadine	Clarinex	Nonsedating antihistamine	5-mg tab 2.5-mg, 5-mg dissolving tab 0.5-mg/ml syrup
Desogestrel with ethinyl estradiol	Mircette, Kariva, Desogen, Apri, Ortho-Cept	Oral contraceptive	0.15-mg/0.02-mg tab
Dexamethasone	Decadron, Deltasone	Adrenal corticosteroid	0.25-mg, 0.5-mg, 0.75-mg, 1-mg, 1.5-mg, 2-mg, 4-mg, 6-mg tab 0.5-mg/5-ml, 0.5-mg/0.5-ml oral soln 0.01%, 0.04% topical aerosol
Dexmethylphenidate HCl	Focalin, Focalin XR	CNS stimulant	2.5-mg, 5-mg, 10-mg tab 5-mg, 10-mg, 20-mg ER cap
Diazepam (CIV)	Valium	Benzodiazepine (anticonvulsant)	2-mg, 5-mg, 10-mg tab 1-mg/ml, 5-mg/ml, 5-mg/5-ml oral soln 5-mg/ml inj 2.5-mg, 5-mg, 10-mg, 15-mg, 20-mg rectal gel
Diclofenac sodium	Voltaren, Voltaren XR	NSAID	75-mg tab 100-mg XR tab

GENERIC NAME	BRAND NAME	CLASS	STRENGTH/DOSAGE FORM
Dicyclomine HCl	Bentyl	Anticholinergic (GI antispasmodic)	10-mg, 20-mg cap 20-mg tab 10-mg/5-ml syrup 10-mg/ml inj
Digoxin	Lanoxin, Digitek, Lanoxicaps	Antiarrythmic Class IV (cardiac glycoside)	0.05-mg, 0.1-mg, 0.2-mg cap 0.125-mg, 0.25-mg, 0.5-mg tab 0.05-mg/ml elixir 0.25-mg/ml, 0.1-mg/ml inj
Diltiazem HCl	Cardizem, Cardizem (SR, CD, LA), Tiazac, Cartia XT	Calcium channel blocker (antihypertensive, antianginal)	30-mg, 60-mg, 90-mg, 120-mg tab 120-mg, 180-mg, 240-mg SR tab 60-mg, 90-mg, 120-mg, 180-mg, 240-mg, 300-mg, 360-mg SR cap 120-mg, 180-mg, 240-mg, 300-mg, 360-mg, 420-mg ER tab 25-mg, 50-mg inj
Diphenoxylate HCl with atropine sulfate (CV)	Lomotil	Antidiarrheal	2.5-mg/0.025-mg tab 2.5-mg/0.025-mg-per-ml liq
Divalproex sodium	Depakote, Depakote ER	Anticonvulsant, antipsychotic	125-mg, 250-mg, 250-mg tab 250-mg, 500-mg ER tab 125-mg sprinkle cap
Docusate sodium	Colace	Stool softener	100-mg tab 50-mg, 100-mg, 240-mg, 250-mg cap 50-mg/15-ml, 60-mg/15-ml, 150-mg/15-ml syrup
Donepezil HCl	Aricept	Acetylcholinesterase inhibitor (Alzheimer's agents)	5-mg, 10-mg tab and disintegrating tab
Dorzolamide HCl with timolol maleate	Cospot	Carbonic anhydrase inhibitor and nonselective beta blocker (anti-glaucoma)	20-mg/5-ml per ml ophth sol
Doxazosin mesylate	Cardura, Cardura XL	Alpha-1 antagonist (antihypertensive, BPH agent)	1-mg, 2-mg, 4-mg, 8-mg tab
Doxepin HCl	Sinequan	Tricyclic antidepressant	10-mg, 25-mg, 50-mg, 75-mg, 100-mg, 150-mg cap 10-mg/ml oral conc
Doxycycline hyclate	Vibramycin, Vibra-Tabs	Tetracycline antibiotic	50-mg, 75-mg, 100-mg cap and tab 200-mg inj
Drospirenone and ethinyl estradiol	Yasmin, Yaz	Oral contraceptive	3-mg/0.02-mg tab
Duloxetine HCl	Cybalta	Antidepressant (serotonin-norepinephrine reuptake inhibitor)	20-mg, 30-mg, 60-mg cap
Dutasteride	Avodart	5-alpha reductase inhibitor (prostate anti-inflammatory)	0.5-mg cap

(Continued)

GENERIC NAME	BRAND NAME	CLASS	STRENGTH/DOSAGE FORM
Enalapril maleate	Vasotec	ACE inhibitor (antihypertensive)	2.5-mg, 5-mg, 10-mg, 20-mg tab 1.25-mg/ml inj 1-mg/ml susp
Erythromycin	Ery-Tab, Erythrocin	Macrolide antibiotic	250-mg, 333-mg, 500-mg tab and cap 2% topical soln, gel, ointment 5% ophth oint
Escitalopram	Lexapro	SSRI (antidepressant)	5-mg, 10-mg, 20-mg tab 5-mg/5-ml liquid
Esomeprazole magnesium	Nexium	PPI (gastric antisecretory)	20-mg, 40-mg cap 20-mg, 40-mg inj
Estradiol (topical)	Vivelle-Dot	Estrogen derivative (hormone replacement)	0.025-mg, 0.0375-mg, 0.05-mg, 0.06-mg, 0.075-mg, 0.1-mg patch 14-mcg/24-h patch 25-mcg vaginal tab 2-mg vaginal ring 0.1-mg vaginal cream
Estradiol (oral)	Estrace	Estrogen derivative	0.5-mg, 1-mg, 2-mg tab
Estrogens (conjugated)	Premarin	Estrogen derivative	0.3-mg, 0.45-mg, 0.625-mg, 0.9-mg, 1.25-mg, 2.5-mg tab 25-mg inj 0.625-mg vaginal cream
Estrogens (conjugated) with medroxyprogesterone acetate	Prempro	Estrogen/progestin combination	0.3-mg/1.5-mg, 0.45-mg/1.5-mg, 0.625-mg/2.5-mg, 0.625-mg/5-mg tab
Eszopiclone (CIV)	Lunesta	Non-BZD hypnotic	1-mg, 2-mg, 3-mg tab
Etodolac	Lodine, Lodine XL	NSAID	400-mg, 500-mg tab 200-mg, 300-mg cap 400-mg, 500-mg, 600-mg SR tab
Etonogestrel and ethinyl estradiol	NuvaRing	Contraceptive	11.7-mg/2.7-mg per vaginal ring
Exenatide	Byetta	Antidiabetic agent (incretin mimetic)	25-mg tab
Ezetimibe	Zetia	Antihyperlipidemic	10-mg tab
Ezetimibe with simvastatin	Vytorin	Antihyperlipidemic	10-mg/10-mg, 10-mg/20-mg, 10-mg/40-mg, 10-mg/80-mg tab
Famotidine	Pepcid	H2 antagonist (antiulcer agent)	10-mg, 20-mg, 40-mg tab 40-mg/5-ml susp 10-mg/ml, 20-mg/50-ml inj
Felodipine	Plendil	Antihypertensive (CCB)	2.5-mg, 5-mg, 10-mg SR tab
Fenofibrate	Tricor	Antihyperlipidemic agent	48-mg, 50-mg, 154-mg, 160-mg tab 43-mg, 50-mg, 67-mg, 87-mg, 100-mg, 134-mg, 150-mg, 160-mg, 200-mg cap
Fentanyl (transdermal) (CII)	Duragesic	Narcotic analgesic, general anasthetic	0.05-mg/ml inj 100-mcg, 200-mcg, 300-mcg, 400-mcg lozenge 200-mcg, 400-mcg, 600-mcg, 800-mcg, 1200-mcg, 1600-mcg lozenge on a stick 12-mcg/h, 25-mcg/h, 50-mcg/h, 75-mcg/h, 100-mcg/h transdermal patch

GENERIC NAME	BRAND NAME	CLASS	STRENGTH/DOSAGE FORM
Ferrous sulfate	Feosol, Slow Fe	Electrolyte supplement (iron)	167-mg, 200-mg, 324-mg, 325-mg tab 160-mg SR tab and cap 90-mg/5-ml syrup 220-mg/5-ml elixir 75-mg/0.6-ml drops
Fexofenadine HCl	Allegra	Antihistamine (nonsedating)	30-mg, 60-mg, 180-mg tab 60-mg cap
Fexofendine HCl with pseudoephedrine HCl	Allegra-D	Antihistamine/ decongestant	60-mg/120-mg tab
Finasteride	Proscar	Antiandrogen (prostate anti-inflammatory)	1-mg, 5-mg tab
Fluconazole	Diflucan	Antifungal agent	50-mg, 100-mg, 150-mg, 200-mg tab 10-mg/ml, 40-mg/ml susp 2-mg/ml inj
Fluocionide (topical)	Lidex	Coritosteroid (topical) (anti-inflammatory)	0.05% cream
Fluoxetine	Prozac	Antidepressant (SSRI)	10-mg tab 10-mg, 20-mg cap 20-mg/5-ml sol 90-mg SR cap
Fluticasone propionate (nasal)	Flonase	Corticosteroid (intranasal) (antiallergy agent)	50-mcg nasal spray
Fluticasone propionate MDI	Flovent	Corticosteroid (inhalant–oral) (antiasthmatic)	44-mcg, 110-mcg, 220-mg inhalation aerosol
Fluticasone propionate with salmeterol xinafoate	Advair	Antiasthmatic (corticosteroid + long-acting beta$_2$ agonist)	100-mcg/50-mcg, 250-mcg/50-mcg, 500-mcg/50-mcg inhalation powder
Folic acid	Folacin, folate, pteroylglutamine acid	Water-soluble vitamin	1-mg tab 5-mg/ml inj
Fosinopril sodium	Monopril	ACE inhibitor (antihypertensive)	10-mg, 20-mg, 40-mg tab
Furosemide	Lasix	Loop diuretic	20-mg, 40-mg, 80-mg tab 10-mg/ml, 40-mg/5ml oral soln 10-mg/ml inj
Gabapentin	Neurontin	Antiepileptic, anticonvulsant	100-mg, 300-mg, 400-mg cap 100-mg, 300-mg, 400-mg, 600-mg, 800-mg tab 250-mg/5-ml soln
Gatifloxacin (ophthalmic)	Zymar	Antibiotic (quinolone)	200-mg, 400-mg tab 0.3% ophth soln
Gemfibrozil	Lopid	Antihyperlipidemic (fibric acid)	600-mg tab
Glimepiride	Amaryl	Antidiabetic (sulfonylurea)	1-mg, 2-mg, 4-mg tab
Glipizide	Glucotrol, Glucotrol XL	Antidiabetic (sulfonylurea)	5-mg, 10-mg tab 5-mg, 10-mg SR tab

(Continued)

GENERIC NAME	BRAND NAME	CLASS	STRENGTH/DOSAGE FORM
Glyburide	Micronase, Diabeta	Antidiabetic (sulfonylurea)	1.25-mg, 2.5-mg, 5-mg tab 1.5-mg, 3-mg, 4.5-mg, 6-mg micronized tab
Glyburide with metformin HCl	Glucovance	Antidiabetic (sulfonylurea and biguanide)	1.25-mg/250-mg, 2.5-mg/50-mg, 5-mg/500-mg tab
Hydralazine	Apresoline	Antihypertensive (vasodilator)	10-mg, 25-mg, 50-mg, 100-mg tab 20-mg/ml vial
Hydrocodone bitartrate with acetaminophen (CIII)	Lortab, Vicodin, Lorcet, Norco	Opioid analgesic combination	2.5-mg/500-mg, 5-mg/500-mg, 7.5-mg/500-mg, 10-mg/500-mg tab 7.5-mg/500-mg per 15-ml soln
Hydrocodone bitartrate with ibuprofen (CIII)	Vicoprofen	Opioid analgesic combination	7.5-mg/200-mg tab
Hydrocortisone valerate	Westcort	Corticosteroid (topical anti-inflammatory)	0.2% cream and ointment
Hydroxychloroquine sulfate	Plaquenil	Antimalarial (aminoquinoline)	200-mg tab
Hydroxyzine HCl	Atarax	First-generation antihistamine (antianxiety, antipruritic)	10-mg, 25-mg, 50-mg tab 10-mg/5-ml syrup 25-mg/5-ml susp 25-mg/ml, 50-mg/ml inj
Hyoscyamine sulfate	Levsin, Levbid, Levsinex	Anticholinergic (GI antispasmodic, antisecretic)	0.125-mg, 0.15-mg tab 0.125-mg SL tab and disintegrating tab 0.375 SR cap 0.125-mg/ml oral soln 0.125-mg/5-ml elixir 0.5-mg/ml inj
Ibandronate sodium	Boniva	Bisphosphonate derivative (osteoporotic agent)	2.5-mg daily tab 150-mg monthly tab
Ibuprofen	Motrin	NSAID	2.5-mg, 150-mg tab
Indapamide	Lozol	Thiazide-related diuretic	1.25-mg, 2.5-mg tab
Indomethacin	Indocin	NSAID	25-mg, 50-mg cap 75-mg SR cap 25-mg/5-ml oral susp 50-mg supp 1-mg inj
Insulin	Humulin, Novolin	Insulin (antidiabetic)	100 unit/ml inj
Insulin aspart, rDNA origin	Novolog	Insulin (antidiabetic)	100 unit/ml inj
Insulin glargine, rDNA origin	Lantus	Insulin (antidiabetic)	100 unit/ml inj 3-ml cartridge
Insulin lispro, rDNA origin	Humalog	Insulin (antidiabetic)	100 units/ml
Ipratropium bromide with albuterol sulfate (MDI)	Combivent	Antiasthmatic–bronchodilator (anticholinergic and beta$_2$ agonist)	Inhalation aerosol

GENERIC NAME	BRAND NAME	CLASS	STRENGTH/DOSAGE FORM
Ipratropium bromide with albuterol sulfate	Duoneb	Antiasthmatic–bronchodilator (anticholinergic and beta$_2$ agonist)	0.5-mg/3-mg per 3-ml inhalation soln
Irbesartan	Avapro	ARB (angiotensin II receptor blocker)	75-mg, 150-mg, 300-mg tab
Irbesartan with hydrochlorothiazide	Avalide	Antihypertensive (ARB and thiazide diuretic)	150-mg/12.5-mg, 300-mg/12.5-mg, 300-mg/25-mg tab
Isosorbide mononitrate	Imdur	Antianginal (vasodilator)	10-mg, 20-mg tab 30-mg, 60-mg, 120-mg SR tab
Ketoconazole	Nizoral	Antifungal (oral, topical)	200-mg tab 2% cream and shampoo
Lactulose	Chronulac	Osmotic laxative, ammonium detoxicant	10-g/15-ml soln and syrup
Lamotrigine	Lamictal	Anticonvulsant, antiepileptic	25-mg, 100-mg, 150-mg, 200-mg tab 2-mg, 5-mg, 25-mg chewable tab
Lansoprazole	Prevacid	PPI (antisecretory)	15-mg, 30-mg SR cap 15-mg, 30-mg disintegrating tab 15-mg, 30-mg packets for susp 30-mg inj
Latanoprost	Xalatan	Ophthalmic antiglaucoma agent, prostaglandin	0.005% soln
Levalbuterol HCl	Xopenex	Antiasthmatic (beta$_2$ agonist)	0.63-mg/3-ml, 1.25-mg/3-ml inhalation soln
Levetiracetam	Keppra	Anticonvulsant	250-mg, 500-mg, 750-mg tab 100-mg/ml soln
Levofloxacin	Levaquin	Quinolone antibiotic, respiratory floroquinolone	250-mg, 500-mg, 750-mg tab 25-mg/ml soln 25-mg/ml inj 0.5%, 1.5% ophth soln
Levonorgestrel with ethinyl estradiol	Alesse, Aviane	Oral contraceptive (estrogen and progestin combination)	0.1-mg/0.02-mg tab
Levonorgestrel with ethinyl estradiol (triphasic)	Trivora, Triphasil, Enpresse	Oral contraceptive (estrogen and progestin combination)	28-tab cycle packet
Levothyroxine sodium	Synthroid, Levoxyl, Levothroid	Thyroid hormone	25-mcg, 50-mcg, 75-mcg, 88-mcg, 100-mcg, 112-mcg, 125-mcg, 137-mcg, 150-mcg, 175-mcg, 200-mcg, 300-mcg tab
Lidocaine (transdermal)	Lidoderm	Topical analgesic	5% patch
Lisinopril	Prinvil, Zestril	ACE inhibitor (antihypertensive)	2.5-mg, 5-mg, 10-mg, 20-mg, 30-mg, 40-mg tab
Lisinopril with hydrochlorothiazide	Zestoretic, Prinzide	Antihypertensive (ACE inhibitor and thiazide diuretic combo)	10-mg/12.5-mg, 20-mg/12.5-mg, 20-mg/25-mg tab

(Continued)

GENERIC NAME	BRAND NAME	CLASS	STRENGTH/DOSAGE FORM
Lithium carbonate	Lithonate, Lithotabs, Lithobid	Antipsychotic	150-mg, 300-mg, 600-mg, cap 300-mg, 450-mg SR tab
Lorazepam (CIV)	Ativan	BZD (antianxiety agent)	0.5-mg, 1-mg, 2-mg tab 2-mg/ml soln 2-mg/ml, 4-mg/ml inj
Losartan potassium	Cozaar	Angiotensin II receptor blocker (ARB), antihypertensive	25-mg, 50-mg tab
Losartan potassium with hydrochlorothiazide	Hyzaar	Antihypertensive (ARB and thiazide diuretic)	50-mg/12.5-mg, 100-mg/12.5-mg, 100-mg/25-mg tab
Lovastatin	Mevacor	Antihyperlipidemic (HMG-CoA reductase inhibitor)	10-mg, 20-mg, 40-mg, tab 10-mg, 20-mg, 40-mg, 60-mg ER tab
Meclizine HCl	Antivert	Antivertigo agent, first-generation antihistamine, antiemetic	12.5-mg, 25-mg, 50-mg tab 25-mg, 30-mg cap
Medroxyprogesterone acetate	Provera	Progestin hormone, contraceptive	2.5-mg, 5-mg, 10-mg tab 104-mg/0.65-ml, 150-mg/ml, 400-mg/ml inj
Meloxicam	Mobic	NSAID	7.5-mg tab
Memantine HCl	Namenda	Angent for Alzheimer's (NMDA receptor antagonist)	5-mg, 10-mg, tab 2-mg/ml soln
Mesalamine	Asacol	GI anti-inflammatory (5-aminosalicylic acid derivative)	250-mg CR cap 400-mg delayed-release tab 500-mg supp 4-g/60-ml rectal susp
Metaxalone	Skelaxin	Skeletal-muscle relaxant	800-mg tab
Methadone (CII)	Dolophine, Methadose	Opioid analgesic	5-mg, 10-mg, 40-mg tab 1-mg/ml, 2-mg/ml, 10-mg/ml soln 10-mg/ml inj
Methocarbamol	Robaxin	Skeletal-muscle relaxant	500-mg, 750-mg tab 100-mg/ml inj
Methotrexate	Rheumatrex Dose Pack, Trexall	Antineoplastic agent, antimetabolite (antifolate), DMRD (disease-modiying anti-rheumatic drug)	2.5-mg tab 2.5-ml/ml, 25-mg/ml inj
Methylphenidate HCl (CII)	Concerta Ritalin (SR, LA), Methylin (ER), Metadate CD, Metadate ER	CNS stimulant (ADHD agent)	5-mg, 10-mg, 20-mg tab 2.5-mg, 5-mg, 10-mg chewable tab 5-mg/5-ml, 10-mg/5-ml soln 10-mg, 20-mg, 30-mg, 40-mg SR cap 10-mg, 18-mg, 20-mg, 27-mg, 36-mg, 54-mg SR tab 10-mg, 15-mg, 20-mg, 30-mg transdermal patch

GENERIC NAME	BRAND NAME	CLASS	STRENGTH/DOSAGE FORM
Methylprednisolone	Medrol	Systemic corticosteroid, anti-inflammatory agent	2-mg, 4-mg, 8-mg, 16-mg, 24-mg, 32-mg tab
Metoclopramide HCl	Reglan	Antiemetic, prokinetic GI agent	5-mg, 10-mg tab 5-mg/5-ml soln 5-mg/ml inj
Metolazone	Zaroxolyn	Thiazide-related diuretic	2.5-mg, 5-mg, 10-mg tab
Metoprolol succinate	Toprol-XL	Antihypertensive (beta blocker, beta-1 selective)	25-mg, 50-mg, 100-mg, 200-mg ER tab
Metoprolol tartrate	Lopressor	Antihypertensive (beta blocker, beta-1 selective)	50-mg, 100-mg tab 5-mg/5-ml ampoule
Metronidazole	Flagyl, Flagyl ER	Antibacterial, antiprotozoal, amebicide	250-mg, 500-mg tab 375-mg cap 750-mg SR tab 500-mg inj 0.75% lotion and emulsion 0.75%, 1% cream and gel
Minocycline hydrochlorothiazide	Minocin	Tetracycline antibiotic	50-mg, 75-mg, 100-mg cap and tab 50-mg/5-ml susp 1-mg SR microspheres
Mirtazapine	Remeron	Antidepressant, $alpha_2$ antagonist	15-mg, 30-mg, 45-mg tab and disintegrating tab
Modafinil (CIV)	Provigil	Pseudosympathomimetic (stimulant)	100-mg, 200-mg cap
Mometasone furoate (topical)	Elocon	Corticosteroid (topical anti-inflammatory)	0.1% cream
Mometasone furoate monohydrate (intranasal)	Nasonex	Corticosteroid (antiallergy agent)	50-mcg nasal spray
Monteleukast sodium	Singulair	Antiasthmatic (leukotriene receptor antagonist)	5-mg, 10-mg tab 4-mg chewable tab 4-mg oral granules
Morphine sulfate (extended release) (CII)	MS Contin	Opioid analgesic	15-mg, 30-mg, 60-mg, 100-mg, 200-mg tab
Moxifloxacin HCl (oral)	Avelox, Vigamox	Floroquinolone antibiotic (oral, ophthalmic, respiratory)	400-mg tab 0.5% ophth soln 160-mg/100-ml infusion
Mupirocin	Bactroban	Topical antibiotic	2% ointment and cream
Nabumetone	Relafen	NSAID	500-mg, 750-mg tab
Naproxen sodium	Anaprox, Anaprox DS	NSAID	275-mg tab 550-mg DS tab
Naproxen	Aleve, Naprosyn, Midol ER	NSAID	250-mg, 375-mg, 500-mg tab 125-mg/5-ml susp
Niacin	Niaspan	Antihyperlidemic	50-mg, 100-mg, 250-mg, 500-mg tab 125-mg, 250-mg, 400-mg, 500-mg, 750-mg, 1000-mg SR cap

(Continued)

GENERIC NAME	BRAND NAME	CLASS	STRENGTH/DOSAGE FORM
Nifedipine	Procardia, Procardia XL, Nifedical XL, Adalat CC	CCB (antihypertensive, antianginal)	10-mg, 20-mg cap 30-mg, 60-mg, 90-mg SR tab
Nitrofurantoin	Macrodantin, Macrobid	Antibacterial	25-mg/ml susp 25-mg, 50-mg, 100-mg cap
Nitroglycerin	Nitrostat, Nitroquick, Nitrocap, Nitrostat IV, Nitro-Dur, Nitrodisc	Antianginal (vasodilator)	5-mg/ml inj 0.3-mg, 0.4-mg, 0.6-mg sl tab 2.5-mg, 6.5-mg, 9-mg SR tab and cap 0.1-mg/hr, 0.2-mg/hr, 0.3-mg/hr, 0.4-mg/hr, 0.6-mg/hr, 0.8-mg/hr transdermal patch 2% ointment
Norelgestromin and ethinyl estradiol (transdermal)	Ortho Evra	Transdermal contraceptive (estrogen and progestin)	6-mg/0.75-mg transdermal patch
Norethindrone and ethinyl estradiol	Necon 1/35, Ortho Novum 1/35	Oral contraceptive	1-mg/0.035-mg tab
Norethindrone acetate, ethinyl estradiol, and ferrous fumarate	Loestrin 24 FE	Oral contraceptive	24 tabs of 1-mg/20-mcg per pack and 4 tabs of ferrous fumarate
Norgestimate and ethinyl estradiol	Ortho-Cyclen, Sprintec	Oral contraceptive	0.215-mg/0.035-mg tab
Norgestrel and ethinyl estradiol	Ovral, Lo/Ovral, Ogestrel, Cyselle	Oral contraceptive	0.3-mg/0.03-mg tab
Nortriptyline HCl	Pamelor	Tricyclic antidepressant	10-mg, 25-mg, 50-mg, 75-mg cap 10-mg/5-ml soln
Nystatin (oral)	Mycostatin, Nilstat	Antifungal agent	500,000-unit tab 100,000-unit/ml susp 200,000-unit troche 100,000-unit vag tab 100,000 units/g cream, ointment, and powder
Nystatin with Triamcinolone acetonide	Mycolog II	Topical antifungal with topical corticosteroid	100,000 units/1-mg per gram cream and oint
Olanzapine	Zyprexa	Atypical antipsychotic	2.5-mg, 5-mg, 7.5-mg, 10-mg, 15-mg tab 10-mg, 15-mg, 20-mg disintegrating tab 10-mg inj
Olmesartan medexomil	Benicar	Angiotensin II receptor blocker (ARB)—antihypertensive	5-mg, 20-mg, 40-mg tab
Olmesartan medoxomil with hydrochlorothiazide	Benicar-HCT	ARB with thiazide diuretic	20-mg/12.5-mg, 40-mg/12.5-mg, 40-mg/25-mg tab
Olopatadine HCL (ophthalmic)	Patanol	second-generation antihistamine (ophthalmic antiallergy)	0.1% ophth soln
Omega-3-acid ethyl esters	Lovaza	Antihyperlipidemic	1-g cap
Omeprazole	Prilosec	Proton pump inhibitor (PPI)—antiulcer agent	10-mg, 20-mg, 40-mg, cap 20-mg powder for oral susp

GENERIC NAME	BRAND NAME	CLASS	STRENGTH/DOSAGE FORM
Ondansetron HCl	Zofran	Antiemetic (selective 5-HT3 receptor [serotonin] antagonist)	4-mg, 8-mg, 16-mg, 24-mg, tab 4-mg, 8-mg disintegrating tab 4-mg/5-ml oral soln 2-mg/ml, 8-mg/50-ml, 32-mg/50-ml inj
Oseltamivir phosphate	Tamiflu	Antiviral (neuraminidase inhibitor)	75-mg cap 12-mg/ml susp
Oxcarbazepine	Trileptal	Antiepileptic	150-mg, 300-mg, 600-mg tab 300-mg/5-ml susp
Oxybutynin chloride	Ditropan, Ditropan XL	Urinary antispasmodic agent	5-mg tab 5-mg, 10-mg SR tab 5-mg/5-ml syrup 3.9-mg/day transdermal patch
Oxycodone HCl (controlled release) (CII)	OxyContin	Opioid analgesic	10-mg, 20-mg, 40-mg, 80-mg, 160-mg CR tab
Oxycodone with acetaminophen (CII)	Percocet, Roxicet, Endocet	Opioid analgesic	2.5-mg/325-mg, 5-mg/325-mg, 7.5-mg/325-mg, 10-mg/325-mg, 10-mg/650-mg tab
Paroxetine	Paxil	Antidepressant (SSRI)	10-mg, 20-mg, 30-mg, 40-mg tab 12.5-mg, 25-mg, 37.5-mg SR tab 10-mg/5-ml susp
Penicillin V potassium	Veetids, Pen-Vee K, V-Cillin	Penicillin antibiotic	250-mg, 500-mg tab 125-mg/5-ml, 250-mg/5-ml susp
Phenazopyridine HCl	Pyridium	Urinary tract analgesic	95-mg, 97.2-mg, 100-mg, 150-mg, 200-mg tab
Phenobarbital (CIV)	Phenobarbital	Barbiturate anticonvulsant	15-mg, 16-mg, 30-mg, 60-mg, 90-mg, 100-mg tab 16-mg cap 15-mg/5-ml, 20-mg/5-ml liq 30-mg/ml, 60-mg/ml, 65-mg/ml, 130-mg/ml inj
Phentermine HCl	Adipex-P	Weight management (anorexiant; sympathomimetic)	8-mg, 30-mg, 37.5-mg tab 15-mg, 18.75-mg, 30-mg, 37.5-mg cap
Phenytoin sodium	Dilantin	Class Ib antiarrhythmic agent; anticonvulsant	100-mg cap 100-mg, 200-mg, 30-mg SR cap 50-mg chewable tab 125-mg/5-ml susp 50-mg/ml inj
Pioglitazone HCl	Actos	Thiazolidinedione antidiabetic agent	15-mg, 30-mg, 45-mg tab
Piroxicam	Feldene	NSAID	10-mg, 20-mg cap
Polyethylene glycol 3350, NF	Miralax, Glycolax	Laxative osmotic	powder for reconstitution
Potassium chloride	K-Dur, Micro-K, Klor-Con	Potassium supplement	6.7-mEq, 8-mEq, 10-mEq, 20-mEq SR tab 500-mg, 595-mg, tab 20-mEq, 25-mEq, 50-mEq effervescent tab 20-mEq/15-ml, 40-mEq/15-ml, 45-mEq/15-ml liq 15-mEq, 20-mEq, 25-mEq powder 2-mEq/ml inj

(Continued)

GENERIC NAME	BRAND NAME	CLASS	STRENGTH/DOSAGE FORM
Pramipexole dihydrochloride	Mirapex	Anti-Parkinson's agent (dopamine agonist)	0.125-mg, 0.25-mg, 1-mg, 1.5-mg tab
Pravastatin sodium	Pravachol	Antilipemic agent (HMG-CoA reductase inhibitor)	10-mg, 20-mg, 40-mg, 80-mg tab
Prednisolone sodium phosphate	Orapred	Corticosteroid (anti-inflammatory)	5-mg/5-ml liq 0.125%, 1%, 0.9%, 0.11% ophth soln
Prednisone	Deltasone	Corticosteroid (anti-inflammatory)	1-mg, 2.5-mg, 5-mg, 10-mg, 20-mg, 50-mg tab 5-mg/5-ml, 5-mg/ml soln
Pregabalin	Lyrica	Anticonvulsant, antineuralgic	25-mg, 50-mg, 75-mg, 100-mg, 150-mg, 200-mg, 225-mg, 300-mg cap
Prochlorperazine	Compazine	Phenothiazine (typical) antipsychotic, antiemetic	5-mg, 10-mg, 25-mg tab 10-mg, 15-mg, 30-mg SR cap 2.5-mg, 5-mg, 25-mg supp 5-mg/ml inj
Progesterone	Prometrium	Progestin (hormone)	100-mg, 200-mg caps
Promethazine HCl	Phenergan	First-generation antihistamine, antiemetic	12.5-mg, 25-mg, 50-mg tab and supp
Promethazine HCl with codeine phosphate	Phenergan with Codeine	Antihistamine/antitussive	syrup
Propoxyphene napsylate with acetaminophen	Darvocet-N, Darvocet-A	Opioid analgesic, antipyretic	50-mg/325-mg, 100-mg/325-mg tab
Propranolol HCl	Inderal, Inderal LA	Beta blocker (antihypertensive), Class II antiarrythmic agent	10-mg, 20-mg, 40-mg, 60-mg, 80-mg, 90-mg tab 60-mg, 80-mg, 120-mg, 160-mg SR cap 4-mg/ml, 8-mg/ml, 80-mg/ml soln 1-mg/ml inj
Quetiapine fumerate	Seroquel, Seroquel XR	Atypical antipsychotic	25-mg, 100-mg, 200-mg tab
Quinapril	Accupril	ACE inhibitor	5-mg, 10-mg, 20-mg, 40-mg tab
Rabeprazole sodium	Aciphex	Proton pump inhibitor (PPI)	20-mg tab
Raloxifene HCl	Evista	Selective estrogen receptor modulator (SERM), osteoporosis agent	60-mg tab
Ramipril	Altace	ACE inhibitor	1.25-mg, 2.5-mg, 5-mg, 10-mg cap
Ranitidine	Zantac	Histamine (H_2) antagonist	75-mg, 150-mg, 300-mg tab 25-mg, 150-mg effervescent tab 150-mg, 300-mg cap 15-mg/ml syrup 1-mg/ml, 25-mg/ml inj
Risedronate sodium	Actonel	Bisphosphonate derivative (osteoporosis agent)	5-mg, 30-mg, 35-mg tab

GENERIC NAME	BRAND NAME	CLASS	STRENGTH/DOSAGE FORM
Risperidone	Risperdal	Atypical antipsychotic agent, antimanic agent	0.25-mg, 0.5-mg, 1-mg, 2-mg, 3-mg, 4-mg tab 0.5-mg, 1-mg, 2-mg quick-dissolving tab 1-mg/ml soln 25-mg, 37.5-mg, 50-mg inj
Ropinirole HCl	Requip, Requip XL	Anti-Parkinson's agent (dopamine agonist)	0.25-mg, 0.5-mg, 1-mg, 2-mg, 5-mg tab
Rosiglitazone maleate	Avandia	Thiazolidinedione (antidiabetic agent)	2-mg, 4-mg, 8-mg tab
Rosuvastatin calcium	Crestor	HMG-CoA reductase inhibitor (antihyperlipidemic)	5-mg, 10-mg, 20-mg 40-mg tab
Sertraline HCl	Zoloft	SSRI (selective serotonin reuptake inhibitor), Antidepressant	25-mg, 50-mg, 100-mg tab 20-mg/ml liq
Sildenafil citrate	Viagra	Erectile dysfunction agent (phophodiesterase inhibitor)	20-mg, 25-mg, 50-mg, 100-mg tab
Simvastatin	Zocor	HMG-CoA reductase inhibitor	5-mg, 10-mg, 20-mg, 40-mg, 80-mg tab
Sitagliptin phosphate	Januvia	Antidiabetic agent (DPP-4 inhibitor)	25-mg, 50-mg, 100-mg tab
Solifenacin succinate	Vesicare	Anticholinergic agent (urinary bladder modifier)	5-mg, 10-mg tab
Trimethoprim–Sulfamethoxazole	Bactrim, Septra	Sulfonamide derivative antibacterial	80-mg/400-mg, 160-mg/800-mg tab 40-mg/200-mg per 5-ml susp 16-mg/80-mg per 5-ml, 80-mg/400-mg per 5-ml inj
Sumatriptan succinate	Imitrex	Serotonin receptor agonist (antimigrane agent)	25-mg, 50-mg tab 12-mg/ml inj 5-mg, 20-mg nasal spray
Tadalafil	Cialis	Erectile dysfunction agent (phosphodiesterase inhibitor)	5-mg, 10-mg, 20-mg tab
Tamoxifen citrate	Nolvadex	Antineoplastic agent, SERM, estrogen receptor antagonist	10-mg, 20-mg tab
Tamsulosin HCl	Flomax	Prostate anti-inflammatory (alpha$_1$ blocker)	0.4-mg cap
Telmisartan	Micardis	Angiotensin II receptor blocker (ARB)	40-mg, 80-mg tab
Telmisartan with hydrochlorothiazide	Micardis HCT	ARB/thiazide diuretic	40-mg/12.5-mg, 80-mg/12.5-mg, 80-mg/25-mg tab
Temazepam (CIV)	Restoril	Benzodiazepine	7.5-mg, 15-mg, 30-mg cap

(Continued)

GENERIC NAME	BRAND NAME	CLASS	STRENGTH/DOSAGE FORM
Terazosin HCl	Hytrin	Antihypertensive, BPH treatment (alpha adrenergic blocking agent)	1-mg, 2-mg, 5-mg, 10-mg cap
Tetracycline HCl	Sumycin, Panmycin	Tetracycline antibiotic	100-mg, 125-mg, 250-mg, 500-mg cap 125-mg/5-ml susp
Thyroid, dessicated	Armour Thyroid	Thyroid hormone	15-mg, 30-mg, 60-mg 90-mg, 120-mg, 180-mg, 240-mg, 300-mg tab
Tiotropium bromide (inhalation)	Spiriva	Antiasthmatic (anticholinergic agent)	18-mcg cap for inhalation
Tobramycin and dexamethasone (ophthalmic)	TobraDex	Antibiotic, ophthalmic corticosteroid	0.3%/0.1% ophth soln and oint
Tolterodine tartrate	Detrol, Detrol LA	Anticholinergic agent (urinary bladder modifier)	1-mg, 2-mg tab 2-mg, 4-mg SR tab
Topiramate	Topamax	Anticonvulsant	25-mg, 100-mg, 200-mg tab 15-mg, 25-mg, 50-mg cap
Torsemide	Demadex	Loop diuretic	5-mg, 10-mg, 20-mg, 100-mg tab 10-mg/ml inj
Tramadol HCl with acetaminophen	Ultracet	Analgesic	37.5-mg/325-mg tab
Tramadol	Ultram, Ultram ER	Opioid analgesic	50-mg tab and disintegrating tab
Travoprost	Travatan	Antiglaucoma agent (ophthalmic prostaglandin)	0.004% ophth soln
Trazadone	Desyrel	Antidepressant (serotonin reuptake inhibitor)	50-mg, 100-mg, 150-mg, 300-mg tab
Triamcinolone acetonide	Kenalog, Nasacort AQ	Corticosteroid	3-mg/ml, 10-mg/ml, 40-mg/ml inj 100-mcg aerosol 55-mcg inhal 55-mcg spray 0.5-mg/ml nasal spray 0.025%, 0.1%, 0.5% cream, ointment, and lotion 10.3% topical spray
Triamterene with hydrochlorothiazide	Dyazide, Maxzide	Potassium-sparing diuretic/thiazide diuretic	Dyazide: 37.5-mg/25-mg cap Maxzide: 50-mg/75-mg tab
Valacyclovir HCl	Valtrex	Antiviral agent	500-mg cap
Valsartan	Diovan	Angiotensin II receptor blocker (ARB)	40-mg, 80-mg, 160-mg tab
Valsartan with hydrochlorothiazide	Diovan-HCT	ARB/thiazide diuretic	80-mg/12.5-mg, 160-mg/12.5-mg, 160-mg/25-mg, 320-mg/12.5-mg, 320-mg/25-mg tab
Verdanafil HCl	Levitra	Erectile dysfunction agent (phosphodiesterase inhibitor)	2.5-mg, 5-mg, 10-mg, 20-mg tab

GENERIC NAME	BRAND NAME	CLASS	STRENGTH/DOSAGE FORM
Varenicline tartrate	Chantix	Smoking-cessation agent (partial nicotine agent)	0.5-mg, 1-mg cap
Venlafaxine HCl	Effexor, Effexor XR	Antidepressant (serotonin/ norepinephrine reuptake inhibitor)	25-mg, 37.5-mg, 50-mg, 75-mg, 100-mg tab 37.5-mg, 75-mg, 150-mg SR cap
Verapamil HCl	Isoptin, Calan, Verelen	Class 4 antiarrythmic agent, calcium channel blocker (CCB)	40-mg, 80-mg, 120-mg tab 120-mg, 180-mg, 240-mg SR tab 100-mg, 120-mg, 180-mg, 200-mg, 240-mg, 300-mg SR cap 5-mg/2-ml inj
Vitamin D, ergocalciferol	Drisdol	Vitamin	50,000 IU cap
Warfarin sodium (crystalline)	Coumadin	Anticoagulant (vitamin-K antagonist)	1-mg, 2-mg, 2.5-mg, 3-mg, 4-mg, 5-mg, 6-mg, 7.5-mg, 10-mg tab 2.5-mg/ml inj
Ziprasidone HCl	Geodon	Atypical antipsychotic	20-mg, 40-mg, 60-mg, 80-mg cap 20-mg/ml inj 10-mg/ml susp
Zolpidem tartrate (CIV)	Ambien, Ambien CR	Hypnotic sedative (nonbenzodiazepine)	5-mg, 10-mg, tab 6.25-mg, 12/5-mg ER tab

When selecting a drug off the shelf, it is a good practice to read the label at least three times: Once when the drug is pulled, once when the drug is filled, and again when the drug is returned to the stock shelf. By doing this, the pharmacy technician can help the pharmacy reduce medication errors. Following is a sample listing of sound-alike, look-alike drugs.

Acetohexamide	Acetazolamide	Lamivudine	Lamotrigine
Advicor	Advair	Leukeran	Leucovorin calcium
Amicar	Omacor	MS Contin	OxyContin
Avinza	Evista	Mucinex	Mucomyst
Cardura	Coumadin	Opium tincture	Paregoric (camphorated opium tincture)
Darvocet	Percocet		
Diabeta	Zebeta	Prilosec	Prozac
Diflucan	Diprivan	Retrovir	Ritonavir
Effexor XR	Effexor	Ephedrine	Epinephrine
Folic acid	Leucovorin calcium (folinic acid)	Hydromorphone	Morphine
Heparin	Hespan	Hydroxyzine	Hydralazine
Hydrocodone	Oxycodone	Metformin	Metronidazole
Idarubicin	Doxorubicin; daunorubicin	Vinblastine	Vincristine

As a general guideline, the following auxiliary labels should be used when filling medications in the corresponding drug categories. Always check individual drugs for their specific requirements.

DRUG CATEGORY	AUXILLARY LABEL	INDIVIDUAL DRUGS
Antibiotics	Take on an empty stomach Finish all medications	Penicillin Amoxicillin
Antibiotic, reconstituted susp	Take on an empty stomach Finish all medications before expiration date Refrigerate Expires on:	Amoxicillin Dicloxicillin
Antihistimines, first-generation	May cause drowsiness	Diphenhydramine
Inhalers, oral	Shake well before using	Albuterol Salmeterol
Metronidazole	Do not drink alcohol	Flagyl
Controlled substances	May cause drowsiness Do not drink alcohol	Hydrocodone with aceataminophen Diazepam
NSAIDs	Take with food or milk	Ibuprofen Indomethacin
Phenazopyridine and rifampin	May cause discoloration of urine or feces	Pyridium Rifadin
Ophthalmic drugs	For the EYE	Propine Timoptic
Rectal drugs	For rectal use	Promethazine suppositories
Suspensions	Shake well	Septra Oral Susp Cortisporin Otic Susp
Tetracycline	Do not take with antacids or dairy products May cause photosensitivity Take on an empty stomach Finish all medications	Sumycin Acromycin
Topical drugs	External use only	Hydrocortisone cream Erythromycin topical soln
Vaginal drugs	For vaginal use only	Nystatin vag tabs

SUMMARY

A solid understanding and knowledge of the top 200 drugs is not only necessary for the certification exam, it is paramount to being a quality pharmacy technician. If you have difficulty with this information, make a set of flash cards—then review, review, and review.

Practice Certification Exam I

This practice exam has been designed to simulate the certification exam in both the number and style of questions as well as the content. You should be able to complete this exam within two hours.

1. Calculate the flow rate in drops per minute if a physician orders D5W/NS 1400 ml over 12 hr using an administration set that delivers 40 gtt/ml.
   a. 87 gtt/min
   b. 68 gtt/min
   c. 117 gtt/min
   d. 78 gtt/min

2. The drug enalapril would be categorized into which of the following classification groups?
   a. beta-blocker
   b. ACE inhibitor
   c. NSAID
   d. antiemetic

3. The retail price of a prescription is based on average wholesale price (AWP) plus a dispensing fee. Using the following fee table, calculate the retail price of a prescription for 30 tablets if a bottle of 100 tablets has an AWP of $76.78.

AWP	DISPENSING FEE
$0–$5.00	$4.75
$5.01–$10.00	$5.75
$10.01–$20.00	$6.75
$20.00 and up	$7.75

   a. $13.72
   b. $23.03
   c. $30.78
   d. $32.91

4. Of the following prescription drugs, which cannot be prescribed with refills?
   a. nifedipine
   b. lorazepam
   c. methylphenidate
   d. hydrocodone/acetaminophen

5. A technician answers the phone and the patient calling states that, after taking a medication she received from the pharmacy a few hours earlier, she is not feeling well and would like to know the side effects of the medication. The technician should:

   a. tell the patient the side effects of the medication, since they are commonly known to all pharmacy personnel
   b. put the patient on hold and notify the pharmacist of the situation
   c. ask the patient to hold while he looks up the side effects in a reference book
   d. tell the patient to lie down and maybe the side effects will wear off soon

6. Diphenhydramine is the generic name for which of these drugs?

   a. Benadryl
   b. Dramamine
   c. Bentyl
   d. Soma

7. A local dermatologist has special-ordered 60 g of 1.5% hydrocortisone cream for a patient. The pharmacy has in stock a 2.5% hydrocortisone cream and a 1% hydrocortisone cream. How much of each will the technician need to prepare this compound correctly?

   a. 40 g of 2.5% and 20 g of 1%
   b. 40 g of 1% and 20 g of 2.5%
   c. 30 g of each strength
   d. 45 g of 1% and 15 g of 2.5%

8. Who must initiate an order for an investigational drug for patient use?

   a. a pharmacy director
   b. a pharmacist
   c. a technician
   d. a physician

9. How many 500-mg metronidazole tablets will be needed to compound 150 ml of 3% metronidazole suspension?

   a. 7
   b. 9
   c. 10
   d. 18

10. A medication given to reduce a fever is called:

   a. an analgesic
   b. an antitussive
   c. an anthelmintic
   d. an antipyretic

11. Medications that are prepackaged into unit-dose or unit-of-use containers must have the following information included on the package labeling:

   a. patient's name, dispensing date, name of medication, and directions for use
   b. medication name and strength, lot number, and expiration date
   c. medication name and strength, lot number, and directions for use
   d. directions for use, medication name and strength, and expiration date

12. A patient brings the following prescription into your pharmacy: Amoxil 400 mg po tid for 10 days. Your pharmacy has in stock an Amoxil oral suspension 250 mg/5 ml. What is the exact volume of medication you will need to correctly and completely fill the prescription for the patient?

   a. 150 ml
   b. 168 ml
   c. 240 ml
   d. 200 ml

13. When mixing cytotoxic agents for intravenous use, what type of syringe is required?

   a. glass
   b. Luer-Loc
   c. slip-tip
   d. reusable

14. To what class of controlled substances does Lortab belong?

   a. II
   b. III
   c. IV
   d. V

15. Inventory turnover rate refers to:

   a. how often employees quit and new employees are hired to replace them
   b. how long it takes the pharmacy to process a new prescription
   c. how many times a year shelves are inspected for expired medications
   d. how often medications are used and reordered

16. The portion of the retail price of a prescription that the patient must pay is known as the:

   a. deductible
   b. co-payment
   c. average wholesale price
   d. none of the above

17. How many capsules will it take to completely fill the following prescription: cephalexin 500 mg, i po tid × 14 days?

   a. 14 capsules
   b. 21 capsules
   c. 28 capsules
   d. 42 capsules

18. Prescription medications are often referred to as _____ drugs because of the federal law that requires the packaging to display the following message: "Rx Only."
    a. controlled
    b. legend
    c. prescription
    d. none of the above

19. Stock rotation is the task of making sure that:
    a. the shortest expiration date is in the back
    b. the longest expiration date is in the front
    c. the shortest expiration date is in the front
    d. a and b

20. Which of the following is classified as a beta-blocker?
    a. propranolol
    b. enalapril
    c. verapamil
    d. allopurinol

21. A patient in the hospital needs KCl 8 mEq IV stat. The pharmacy stocks KCl 2 mEq/ml in a 10-mL multidose vial. What is the correct volume to be drawn up?
    a. 2.5 mL
    b. 4 mL
    c. 0.4 mL
    d. 0.04 mL

22. What document is used by the pharmacy to pay the wholesaler for a drug order?
    a. packing slip
    b. invoice
    c. purchase order
    d. DEA Form 222c

23. The pharmacy receives a prescription for 4 oz of 5% ointment. The pharmacy stocks the ointment in strengths of 2% and 10%. To prepare the prescription, how much of each stock ointment is needed?
    a. 50 g of 2% and 70 g of 10%
    b. 12 g of 2% and 108 g of 10%
    c. 75 g of 2% and 45 g of 10%
    d. 45 g of 2% and 75 g of 10%

24. What is the correct temperature for storing an item in the refrigerator?
    a. 2 to 8°C
    b. less than 36°F
    c. 15 to 30°C
    d. 59 to 86°F

25. In an inpatient setting, the pharmacy must receive a direct copy of a physician's order before filling an initial dose. Which of the following is not considered a direct copy?
    a. fax
    b. photocopy
    c. computer-generated transfer
    d. phone call acknowledging the verbal order

26. 300 mL of a Cipro 5% suspension contains how many grams of active ingredient?
    a. 1.5 g
    b. 15 g
    c. 3 g
    d. 30 g

27. The term used to refer to protection of a patient's identity and health information is
    a. motility
    b. confidentiality
    c. mortality
    d. compatibility

28. According to federal law, what is the maximum number of refills permitted for a Schedule III controlled substance?
    a. six refills within one year
    b. three refills within 90 days
    c. five refills within six months
    d. no refills are allowed

29. In the NDC number 69907-3110-01, what does section "3110" identify?
    a. manufacturer
    b. drug product
    c. package size
    d. number of tablets in the bottle

30. The trade name for glipizide is
    a. Diabinese
    b. Micronase
    c. Glucophage
    d. Glucotrol

31. What is the total volume of D5W needed for a 24-hr period if the infusion runs at a rate of 125 ml/hr?
    a. 3000 mL
    b. 1000 mL
    c. 2400 mL
    d. 1250 mL

32. The recommended dose for gentamicin injection is 5 mg/kg/day in three divided doses. If a patient weighs 164 lb, how many milligrams should that patient receive for each dose?
    a. 25 mg
    b. 75 mg
    c. 124 mg
    d. 373 mg

33. Which of the following drugs is classed as an H_2 antagonist?
    a. clonidine
    b. ranitidine
    c. loratadine
    d. clemastine

34. KCl supplements are most often used in combination with:
    a. labetalol
    b. lisinopril
    c. naproxen
    d. furosemide

35. If a patient calls in for refills on Prinivil and Diabeta, which of the following combinations of medications need to be filled for the patient?
    a. lisinopril and glipizide
    b. enalapril and glyburide
    c. enalapril and glipizide
    d. lisinopril and glyburide

36. How much neomycin powder must be added to fluocinolone cream to dispense an order for 60 g of fluocinolone cream with 0.5% neomycin?
    a. 120 mg
    b. 240 mg
    c. 300 mg
    d. 600 mg

37. Which of the sig codes given refers to the following directions: Take two tablets by mouth every 4 to 6 hr as needed?
    a. 2 tabs q4–6h prn
    b. 2 tabs po q4–6h prn
    c. 2 tabs po q4–6h
    d. a or c

38. The pharmacy receives an order for 10% ointment, but it stocks only 5% and 15%. In what ratio would the two stock ointments need to be mixed in order to compound the prescription order correctly?
    a. 1:1
    b. 1:2
    c. 2:1
    d. 1:3

39. Which of the following drugs is most likely to cause photosensitivity?
    a. nifedipine
    b. naproxen
    c. tetracycline
    d. glyburide

40. After reconstitution, how many 250-mg doses of Claforan can be withdrawn from a 2-g vial?
    a. 2 doses
    b. 4 doses
    c. 6 doses
    d. 8 doses

41. A medication that should be protected from exposure to light is
    a. promethazine
    b. tetracycline
    c. erythromycin
    d. nitroglycerin

42. The blower on the laminar airflow workbench should remain on at all times. If it is turned off for any reason, it should remain on for at least _____ before being used to prepare IV admixtures and other products.
    a. 15 minutes
    b. 1 hour
    c. 30 minutes
    d. 45 minutes

43. Which of the following needle sizes has the largest bore?
    a. 23 gauge
    b. 18 gauge
    c. 27 gauge
    d. 29 gauge

44. When metronidazole is dispensed for a patient, which auxiliary label should be affixed to the dispensing container?
    a. No alcohol
    b. No dairy products
    c. Take with food or milk
    d. May cause drowsiness

45. If 500 mL of a 15% solution is diluted to 1500 mL, how would you label the final strength of the solution?
    a. 20%
    b. 5%
    c. 0.05%
    d. 0.20%

46. A prescription reading "iii gtt a.s. tid prn pain" should have which set of directions printed on the dispensing label?
    a. Instill 3 drops in the left eye three times daily as needed for pain.
    b. Instill 3 drops in the left ear three times daily as needed for pain.
    c. Instill 3 drops in the right ear two times daily as needed for pain.
    d. Instill 3 drops in the right eye three times daily as needed for pain.

47. A patient with a penicillin allergy is most likely to exhibit a sensitivity to:
    a. tetracycline
    b. erythromycin
    c. cefaclor
    d. gentamicin

48. A Tylenol #3 tablet contains 30 mg of codeine. The amount of codeine is also equivalent to:
    a. $\frac{1}{4}$ gr
    b. $\frac{1}{2}$ gr
    c. 1 gr
    d. 2 gr

49. An IV infusion order is written for 1 L of D5W/0.45% NS to run over 12 hr. The set that will be used delivers 15 gtt/ml. What is the flow rate be in gtt/min?
    a. 7 gtt/min
    b. 21 gtt/min
    c. 25 gtt/min
    d. 125 gtt/min

50. To ensure that it is working properly, the laminar airflow workbench should be inspected by qualified personnel at least:
    a. every six months
    b. every year
    c. every three years
    d. every five years

51. Zovirax and Epivir are both classed as _____ agents.
    a. antimalarial
    b. tuberculosis
    c. antiviral
    d. antifungal

52. A physician writes an order for a patient to receive KCl 40 mEq/1 L NS @ 80 ml/hr. What amount of KCl will the patient receive per hour?
    a. 6.8 mEq
    b. 3.2 mEq
    c. 2.3 mEq
    d. 8.6 mEq

53. Na is the chemical symbol for which of the following elements?
    a. nitrogen
    b. potassium
    c. hydrochloride
    d. sodium

54. When withdrawing medication from an ampoule, what size filter needle will be sufficient to filter out any tiny glass fragments that might have fallen into the solution?

    a. 0.2 micron
    b. 0.5 micron
    c. 2 micron
    d. 5 micron

55. Which of the following conditions is the drug rifampin used to treat?
    a. influenza
    b. tuberculosis
    c. nail fungus
    d. urinary tract infection

56. When measuring liquid in a graduated cylinder, where is the volume of liquid read?
    a. top surface of the liquid
    b. top of the meniscus
    c. center of the meniscus
    d. bottom of the meniscus

57. How many grams of 2% silver nitrate ointment will deliver 1 g of the active ingredient?
    a. 25 g
    b. 4 g
    c. 50 g
    d. 20 g

58. The federal law enacted in 1970 that requires the use of child-resistant safety caps on all dispensing containers unless otherwise desired by the patient is known as the:
    a. Controlled Substances Act
    b. Poison Prevention Act
    c. Pure Food and Drug Act
    d. Harrison Narcotic Act

59. Into what size bottle will a prescription for 180 mL of cough syrup best fit?
    a. 2 oz
    b. 4 oz
    c. 6 oz
    d. 8 oz

60. If a patient should receive a medication at 15 mg/kg/day in three equally divided doses, what will be the approximate dose if the patient weighs 142 lb?
    a. 968 mg
    b. 323 mg
    c. 2904 mg
    d. 284 mg

61. If one of your pharmacy's patients has had an adverse drug reaction, _____ should be used to report it.
    a. the HCFA form
    b. the MedWatch form
    c. DEA Form 222c
    d. the Universal Claim Form

62. Of the following choices, which pair of drugs are H$_2$ antagonists?
    a. Zantac and Prevacid
    b. Prinivil and Tagamet
    c. Pepcid and Zantac
    d. Vasotec and Motrin

63. A pharmacy wants to make a 30% profit on an item that costs $4.50. What would the retail selling price have to be in order to make such a profit?
    a. $6.23
    b. $7.10
    c. $5.85
    d. $6.40

64. Which statement is true concerning the drug tetracycline?
    a. It should be given with food or milk for best absorption.
    b. It should not be given with milk products or antacids for best absorption.
    c. It should be given with milk because it is upsetting to the stomach.
    d. Exposure to sunlight will not affect a patient taking this medication.

65. Under what schedule of controlled substances does the drug temazepam fall?
    a. II
    b. III
    c. IV
    d. V

66. When storing an item at a controlled room temperature, the temperature of the room should be
    a. 2 to 8°C
    b. 36 to 46°F
    c. higher than 30°C
    d. 15 to 30°C

67. A list of medications that a physician may prescribe from within a given institutional setting is called:
    a. an MSDS
    b. a formulary
    c. a closed panel of drugs
    d. an open system

68. Which of the following is considered PHI under HIPAA regulations?
    a. patient address
    b. patient date of birth
    c. patient name
    d. all the above

69. If a vial slips from your hand while you are preparing an IV admixture and breaks on the floor or other surface, a spill kit must be used to clean the area if the vial contained which of the following medications?
    a. ceftriaxone
    b. potassium chloride
    c. amphotericin b
    d. vinblastine

70. During cleaning of the laminar airflow workbench while preparing to making IV admixtures, which of the following statements is true?
    a. The work surface should be cleaned first using a continuous side-to-side motion.
    b. 70% isopropyl alcohol should be sprayed onto the HEPA filter to ensure its cleanliness.
    c. The sides should be cleaned from top to bottom, working outward from the filter.
    d. The sides should be cleaned from top to bottom, working toward the filter.

71. What volume of 5% aluminum acetate solution will be needed if 120 mL of 0.05% solution is extemporaneously compounded for a prescription?
    a. 12 mL
    b. 1.2 mL
    c. 8.3 mL
    d. 0.83 mL

72. Ampicillin powder for injection should be reconstituted with and diluted in _____ for best stability.
    a. D5W
    b. 0.9% sodium chloride
    c. Lactated Ringers
    d. 0.45% sodium chloride

73. How many 1-L bags will be needed if D5W is to run at 60 ml/hr for 20 hr?
    a. one bag
    b. two bags
    c. three bags
    d. four or more bags

74. What document is used by the wholesaler to pull the pharmacy's order from its shelves?
    a. packing slip
    b. invoice
    c. purchase order
    d. DEA Form 222c

75. A pharmacy has 20 mL of a 1:200 solution in stock. If the pharmacist has asked the technician to dilute the solution to 500 mL, what will be the strength of the final product?
    a. 2%
    b. 2.5%
    c. 25%
    d. 0.02%

76. When an antibiotic injection is given in a small volume of solution that is connected to the main line of IV fluids the patient receives, it is commonly known as an:
    a. IV bag
    b. IV injection
    c. IV piggyback
    d. IV push

77. Although state laws differ on record retention, federal law requires that prescription records be kept for _____ year(s).
    a. 1
    b. 5
    c. 2
    d. 7

78. The largest gelatin capsule used for extemporaneous compounding is
    a. 000
    b. 0
    c. 10
    d. 5

79. All manipulations in the laminar airflow workbench should take place at least _____ from within the front edge of the hood.
    a. 4 in.
    b. 6 in.
    c. 8 in.
    d. 10 in.

80. Which of the following drugs is classified as a calcium channel blocker?
    a. amlodipine
    b. atenolol
    c. enalapril
    d. nitroglycerin

81. When using a manual inventory system, items that need to be ordered are written down by all pharmacy personnel. This writing of a list of items that need to be ordered is referred to as:
    a. a purchase order
    b. an invoice
    c. a want book
    d. an MAR

82. Which of the following DEA numbers would not be valid for Dr. Ann Cosgrove?
    a. AC6782329
    b. AC3081421
    c. AC1355672
    d. BC3421234

83. Of all drug recall classes, a _____ recall would not likely cause harm to the patient, because it is the least severe.

    a. Class I
    b. Class II
    c. Class III
    d. Class IV

84. The form used for ordering Schedule II narcotics is known as:
    a. DEA Form 240
    b. DEA Form 222
    c. DEA Form 121
    d. DEA Form 200

85. Which of the following drugs requires special pharmacy handling and ordering?
    a. controlled substances
    b. chemotherapy drugs
    c. investigational drugs
    d. all the above

86. The Orange Book is most often used to find _____.
    a. generic equivalents
    b. direct prices
    c. therapeutic equivalents
    d. manufacturers' standards

87. Nursing station inspections are primarily the responsibility of the:
    a. nurse
    b. pharmacist
    c. pharmacy director
    d. pharmacy technician

88. Which of the following pairs of medications could cause a major drug–drug interaction if taken together by a patient?
    a. hydrocodone and naproxen
    b. warfarin and aspirin
    c. penicillin and trimethoprim
    d. glyburide and metformin

89. A patient takes NPH insulin according to the following dosage regimen: 35 units sq every morning and 15 units every evening. How many vials of insulin U-100 will the patient need for a 30-day supply?
    a. one vial
    b. two vials
    c. three vials
    d. four or more vials

90. Which of the following medications should always be dispensed in a glass container?
    a. aminophylline
    b. dopamine
    c. potassium
    d. nitroglycerin

chapter 9

Practice Certification Exam II

This practice exam has been designed to simulate the certification exam in both the number and style of questions as well as the content. You should be able to complete this exam within two hours.

1. The device used to compound three-in-one total parenteral nutrition solutions is the:
   a. PhaSeal
   b. Automix
   c. Pyxis
   d. MedCarousel

2. A solid dosage form containing active and inactive ingredients and prepared either by compression or molding methods is a:
   a. capsule
   b. tablet
   c. emulsion
   d. paste

3. Atenolol is to Tenormin as Ramipril is to _____.
   a. Accupril
   b. Lyrica
   c. Aciphex
   d. Altace

4. A method used to identify an employee's individual strengths and weaknesses and provide the employer with information relative to the employee's capacity for retention and promotion is the:
   a. personnel checklist
   b. process validation
   c. employee performance appraisal
   d. employee handbook

5. The _____ is used to record what the pharmacy owes its suppliers and other creditors.
   a. accounts payable ledger
   b. accounts receivable ledger
   c. purchases journal
   d. cash receipts journal

6. Mixing calcium gluconate and sodium phosphate together in the same syringe will cause:
   a. precipitation
   b. incompatibility
   c. intolerance
   d. injunction

7. A preparation of finely divided undissolved drugs dispersed in a liquid vehicle is
   a. an elixir
   b. a solution
   c. a syrup
   d. a suspension

8. A _____ is a system in which the item is deducted from inventory as it is sold or dispensed.
   a. turnover
   b. Pyxis
   c. Baker cell
   d. POS system

9. Which of the following OTC drugs is contraindicated for a patient taking warfarin?
   a. diphenhydramine
   b. loratidine
   c. psyllium
   d. aspirin

10. Effective communication in pharmacy practice can be hindered by:
   a. visual impairment
   b. auditory loss
   c. speech impairment
   d. all of the above

11. Which of the following laws requires pharmacists to counsel Medicaid patients?
   a. Controlled Substances Act
   b. Omnibus Budget Reconciliation Act of 1990
   c. Medicare Part D
   d. Health Insurance Portability and Accountability Act

12. A substance or a mixture of substances added to a tablet to facilitate its breakup or disintegration after administration is a:
   a. terminator
   b. disintegrator
   c. binder
   d. diluent

13. A solid dosage form in which the drug substance is enclosed in either a hard or soft soluble container or a shell of a suitable form of gelatin is a:
   a. capsule
   b. pill
   c. tablet
   d. suppository

14. What is the generic name for Effexor?
   a. verdanafil
   b. venlafaxine
   c. verapamil
   d. valacyclovir

15. The only drug approved to treat high blood pressure during pregnancy is
   a. lidocaine
   b. clonidine
   c. metoprolol
   d. methyldopa

16. The only antihypertensive drug available as a transdermal delivery system is
   a. nicotine
   b. clonidine
   c. nitroglycerin
   d. lidocaine

17. From the following information, calculate the amount in grams of cetyl ester wax needed to make 1 lb of cold cream:

cetyl ester wax	12.5 parts
white wax	12.0 parts
mineral oil	56.0 parts
sodium borate	0.5 parts
water	19.0 parts

   a. 56.75 g
   b. 12.5 g
   c. 60 g
   d. 0.125 g

18. The drug of choice for emergency IV therapy for arrhythmias is
   a. lidocaine
   b. sodium bicarbonate
   c. dopamine
   d. adrenalin

19. The most important drug in managing atrial flutter and fibrillation is
   a. digitalis
   b. amlodipine
   c. doxazosin
   d. quinine

20. The antagonist to warfarin is
   a. heparin
   b. phytonadione
   c. methyldopa
   d. penicillin VK

21. The _____ provides guidelines for the recall of devices that could cause serious adverse effects.
   a. Safe Medical Devices Act
   b. Kefauver-Harris Amendment
   c. Durham-Humphrey Amendment
   d. Medical Device Amendment

22. Schedule II drugs are ordered using:
    a. DEA Form 224a
    b. DEA Form 222
    c. DEA Form 363a
    d. DEA Form 510a

23. An imbalance between oxygen supply and oxygen demand in cardiac muscle may produce a condition known as:
    a. congestive heart failure
    b. heartburn
    c. myocardial infarction
    d. angina pectoris

24. From the following information, calculate in kilograms the quantity of miconazole needed to prepare 12 kg of powder:

zinc oxide	1 part
calamine	2 parts
miconazole	1.5 parts
bismuth subgalate	3 parts
talc powder	8 parts

    a. 15.5 kg
    b. 0.097 kg
    c. 1.16 kg
    d. 1.5 kg

25. Patients on thiazide diuretics are frequently told to take supplements of or eat foods that are high in which element?
    a. calcium
    b. sodium
    c. chlorine
    d. potassium

26. Which of the following auxiliary labels is needed on a prescription for tetracycline?
    a. take with food or milk
    b. may cause drowsiness
    c. do not drink alcohol
    d. may cause photosensitivity

27. When entering a prescription into the computer, the technician uses T1T3 for the directions "Take 1 tablet by mouth 3 times daily." T1T3 is an example of a(n):
    a. pharmaceutical abbreviation
    b. national drug code
    c. bar code
    d. sig code

28. If state and federal guidelines are different on how long a pharmacy should retain its records, the pharmacy should:
    a. always follow the federal guidelines
    b. always follow the state guidelines
    c. follow the guideline that requires the records to be kept for the shortest period of time
    d. follow the guideline that requires the records to be kept for the longest period of time

29. A pharmacy technician dilutes a 1-g vial of cefazolin with 9.6 ml of sterile water. The resulting solution has a concentration of 100 mg/ml. How much solution should be drawn up for a 500-mg dose?
    a. 4.8 ml
    b. 3 ml
    c. 10 ml
    d. 5 ml

30. How much sucralfate 1 gm/10 ml is required for a dose of 600 mg?
    a. 0.06 ml
    b. 0.6 ml
    c. 6 ml
    d. 60 ml

31. In pharmacies, how can controlled substances be stored?
    a. Controlled substances can be stored in an unlocked cabinet.
    b. Controlled substances can be stored in a securely locked, substantially constructed cabinet.
    c. Controlled substances (Schedule III through V) can be stored on the pharmacy shelves among noncontrolled substances in a manner designed to deter theft.
    d. either b or c

32. _____ is a drug agent extracted from cattle lung.
    a. Proventil HFA
    b. Survanta
    c. Bonine
    d. Serevent

33. Patients taking _____ should always be warned NOT to consume alcohol.
    a. metronidazole
    b. tetracycline
    c. albuterol
    d. prednisone

34. The _____ was a direct result of the thalidomide disaster and made manufacturers more accountable for their products.
    a. Comprehensive Drug Abuse Prevention and Control Act
    b. Medical Device Amendment
    c. Durham-Humphrey Amendment
    d. Kefauver-Harris Amendment

35. Patients should be advised not to drink milk or eat dairy products while taking:
    a. calcium carbonate
    b. tetracycline
    c. penicillin
    d. calciferol

36. Patients should be advised to drink plenty of water and to avoid the sun while taking:
    a. TMP-SMZ
    b. cephalexin
    c. propranolol
    d. warfarin

37. _____ are a class of pharmaceutical agents that kill or inhibit the growth of infection-causing microorganisms.
    a. anesthetics
    b. antilipidemics
    c. antibiotics
    d. antihistamines

38. When a drug recall is issued, which of the following information is listed on the recall along with the drug name and strength?
    a. NDC
    b. lot number
    c. expiration date
    d. distribution date

39. When liquid medications are repackaged into oral syringes, the syringe must:
    a. not be amber in color
    b. be sterile
    c. not be able to accept a needle
    d. be made of glass

40. The agency that oversees the Controlled Substances Act is the:
    a. State Board of Pharmacy
    b. American Society of Health System Pharmacists
    c. Food and Drug Administration
    d. Drug Enforcement Agency

41. If a medication is taken "p.c.," it will be taken:
    a. before meals
    b. around the clock
    c. after meals
    d. with meals

42. All of the following are true statements except:
    a. All controlled substances must be inventoried on the day the pharmacy first dispenses controlled substances.
    b. The inventory of Schedule II medications requires an exact count or measure, while other schedules may be estimated.

c. Prescriptions are the primary records for the acquisition of controlled substances by a pharmacy.
    d. The beginning inventory plus all acquisitions minus dispensing by prescriptions or to other practitioners should equal the current inventory count.

43. A _____ drug is active against both gram-positive and gram-negative bacteria.
    a. neg-gram
    b. bacteriostatic
    c. broad-spectrum
    d. narrow-spectrum

44. A patient weighs 165 lb. How many kilograms does the patient weigh?
    a. 165,000 kg
    b. 75 kg
    c. 363 kg
    d. 330 kg

45. Which of the following vitamins is a fat-soluble vitamin?
    a. thiamine
    b. pyridoxine
    c. cyanocobalamine
    d. phytonadione

46. If an insurance company only pays for a 14 day supply and the prescription is for "i-ii po q4-6h," what is the maximum number of tablets that can be dispensed?
    a. 56
    b. 84
    c. 168
    d. 224

47. Which of the following dosage forms will best mask the bad taste of a drug?
    a. suspension
    b. sublingual tablet
    c. chewable tablet
    d. gel-cap

48. The pharmacy receives an order for lidocaine 2 g in 250 ml of D5W to be infused at 1.5 mg/min. What is the flow rate in ml/hr?
    a. 11 ml/hr
    b. 22 ml/hr
    c. 33 ml/hr
    d. 44 ml/hr

49. Another term used to describe insulin-dependent diabetes is
    a. non–insulin-dependent diabetes
    b. Type I diabetes
    c. Type II diabetes
    d. diabetes insipidus

50. Oral contraceptives interact with:
    a. antibiotics
    b. anticonvulsants
    c. antifungals
    d. all of the above

51. The pharmacy stocks potassium chloride in 20-mEq vials. The concentration of each vial is 2 mEq/ml. How many milliliters are needed for a 30-mEq dose?
    a. 2 ml
    b. 15 ml
    c. 20 ml
    d. 30 ml

52. The maximum allowable cost that an insurer will pay per tablet or dispensing unit for a given product is the:
    a. co-payment
    b. deductible
    c. U&C
    d. MAC

53. Estrogen is contraindicated with:
    a. migraines
    b. smokers
    c. thrombosis history
    d. all of the above

54. A substance with a high potential for abuse that has no currently accepted medical use in the United States and for which there is a lack of accepted safety for use would be classified as:
    a. C-I
    b. C-II
    c. C-III
    d. C-IV

55. What is the percentage strength of a solution if 1 gallon contains 150 grams of active ingredient?
    a. 0.396%
    b. 1%
    c. 1.5%
    d. 3.96%

56. The Anabolic Steroids Act of 1990 placed anabolic steroids into which controlled-substance category?
    a. C-II
    b. C-III
    c. C-IV
    d. C-V

57. The _____ requires that most prescription drugs be dispensed in a childproof container.
    a. Poison Prevention Act
    b. Safe Medical Devices Act
    c. Prescription Drug Marketing Act
    d. Medical Device Amendment

58. _____ should be taken with 8 oz of water before the first food of the day, and the patient must avoid lying down for at least 30 minutes after taking it.
    a. Miacalcin
    b. Didronel
    c. Fosamax
    d. hydrocortisone

59. Digoxin is classified as:
    a. an antihypertensive
    b. a calcium channel blocker
    c. an ACE inhibitor
    d. a cardiac glycoside

60. If a patient is allergic to opioids, he should avoid taking:
    a. acetaminophen
    b. morphine
    c. aspirin
    d. penicillin

61. Which of the following is used to induce labor contractions?
    a. epinephrine
    b. serotonin
    c. dopamine
    d. oxytocin

62. A medication that is used to manage high blood pressure is an:
    a. antitussive
    b. antihypertensive
    c. antipyretic
    d. antibiotic

63. The _____ prohibits the sale of drug samples and reimportation of prescriptions and establishes fair pricing guidelines.
    a. Orphan Drug Act
    b. Prescription Drug Marketing Act
    c. Durham-Humphrey Amendment
    d. Kefauver-Harris Amendment

64. A decrease in susceptibility to a drug's effects from continued use is known as:
    a. addiction
    b. synergism
    c. sensitivity
    d. tolerance

65. Which of the following DEA numbers is valid?
    a. Dr. Russ   AR123456879
    b. Dr. Black   AB56897
    c. Dr. Jones   AJ1234563
    d. Dr. Smith   CS2468217

66. Which of the following is the agent of choice for accidental poisonings, when induction of vomiting is required?
    a. activated charcoal
    b. demulcents
    c. syrup of ipecac
    d. diphenhydramine elixir

67. Which of the following would provide the technician with the most up-to-date and complete information on how to place an inventory order?
    a. MSDS
    b. OSHA guidelines
    c. Pyxis User Manual
    d. Policy & Procedures Manual

68. The rate at which inventory is used is called:
    a. sales journal
    b. sales volume
    c. turnover
    d. net profit

69. Low blood glucose is known as:
    a. glucosuria
    b. hypoglycemia
    c. polyuria
    d. hyperglycemia

70. Certain controlled substances do not bear the federal caution legend and may be sold without a prescription. These products have small quantities of controlled substances included in them and may be sold if certain requirements are met and the proper records are kept. The restrictions on the sale include the following except:
    a. The sale must be made by the pharmacist or a certified pharmacy technician.
    b. The purchaser must be at least 18 and must either be known to the pharmacist or have substantial identification.
    c. Not more than 8 oz or more than 48 dosage units of any substance containing opium in any 48-hr period may be furnished to the purchaser. Not more than 4 oz or 24 dosage units of any other controlled substance may be sold in any 48-hr period.
    d. Pharmacists must maintain a record of the sale in a bound book.

71. Sources of insulin include all of the following except:
    a. cow
    b. horse
    c. pig
    d. human

72. According to federal law, written prescriptions must contain all of the following information except the:
    a. patient's phone number
    b. physician's phone number
    c. drug name and strength
    d. date written

73. A possible cross-sensitivity to _____ is possible for a patient with a severe allergy to penicillin.
    a. cephalosporins
    b. sulfonamides
    c. macrolides
    d. antihypertensives

74. Convert the ratio strength of 1:5000 to a percent strength.
    a. 0.0002%
    b. 0.002%
    c. 0.02%
    d. 2%

75. The bolded section of the National Drug Code 0001-009-**012** indentifies the:
    a. drug's manufacturer
    b. the drug's name, strength, and dosage form
    c. the package size
    d. both a and c

76. Upon discovery of an expired drug, the pharmacy technician should:
    a. rotate the drug to the front of the stock
    b. destroy the drug
    c. follow the pharmacy P&P regarding expired drugs
    d. call the FDA for disposal of the drug

77. A _____-micron filter is commonly used to filter solutions withdrawn from ampoules.
    a. 0.2
    b. 0.5
    c. 2
    d. 5

78. The _____ is a document that contains the goals, policies, and procedures relevant to the employee and the job the employee is assuming.
    a. employee handbook
    b. corporate prospectus
    c. planogram
    d. administration handbook

79. The _____ is used to record the balances that private patients, government agencies, insurance companies, managed-care contractors, and insurers owe the pharmacy.
    a. balance sheet
    b. accounts receivable ledger
    c. cash disbursements journal
    d. sales journal

80. Control of the amount, type, and quality of health care provided to patients within a benefit program is referred to as:
    a. health insurance
    b. managed care
    c. benefit plans
    d. pharmaceutical care

81. 1 pint = _____ ml
    a. 30
    b. 473
    c. 946
    d. 3785

82. The principle that states that patients have the right to full disclosure of all relevant aspects of care and must give explicit consent to treatment before treatment is initiated is
    a. confidentiality
    b. fidelity
    c. informed consent
    d. moral reasoning

83. The provision of drug therapy intended to achieve outcomes that improve the patient's quality of life as it is related to the cure or prevention of a disease, elimination or reduction of a patient's symptoms, or arresting or slowing of a disease process is
    a. pharmaceutical care
    b. managed care
    c. socialized medicine
    d. practice of pharmacy

84. The FDA recall of a product that will cause serious or fatal consequences is classified as:
    a. Class I
    b. Class II
    c. Class III
    d. Class IV

85. Devices:
    a. do not have any restrictions
    b. are defined as instruments, apparatuses, implements, machines, etc.
    c. may be restricted to sale only on the written or oral order of a practitioner licensed to administer such a device
    d. both b and c

86. _____ is a company that buys from the manufacturer and sells to hospitals, pharmacies, and other pharmaceutical dispensers.
    a. The Food and Drug Administration
    b. A wholesaler
    c. A retailer
    d. A mass merchandiser

87. Drugs that are not intended to be sold by a pharmacy, but are intended to promote the sale of that particular drug, are known as:
    a. legend drugs
    b. sample drugs
    c. investigational drugs
    d. over-the-counter drugs

88. The _____ created the legend class of drugs.
    a. Comprehensive Drug Abuse Prevention and Control Act
    b. Medical Device Amendment
    c. Durham-Humphrey Amendment
    d. Kefauver-Harris Amendment

89. Mixing ingredients in order to provide a prescription for a specific patient or a small group of patients is known as:
    a. manufacturing
    b. compressing
    c. compounding
    d. adjudication

90. A prescription is written for 1 lb of 3% salicylic acid in white petrolatum. How many milligrams of salicylic acid are needed?
    a. 13,620 mg
    b. 13.62 mg
    c. 1362 mg
    d. 48 mg

Practice Certification Exam III

This practice test has been designed to simulate the certification exam in the number and style of questions as well as the content. You should be able to complete this exam within two hours.

1. Which route of medication administration is used to inject drugs into muscle?
   a. subq
   b. IV
   c. ID
   d. IM

2. A connection between two or more computer systems that allows for the transfer of data is
   a. an interface
   b. a terminal
   c. a bar code
   d. a window

3. Certification is
   a. the process of granting recognition or vouching for conformance with a standard
   b. the process by which a nongovernmental agency or association grants recognition to an individual who has met certain predetermined qualifications specified by that agency or association
   c. the general process of formally recognizing professional or technical competence
   d. the process of making a list or being enrolled in an existing list

4. An ongoing systematic process for monitoring, evaluating, and improving the quality of pharmacy services is
   a. peer review
   b. quality assurance
   c. process validation
   d. job performance evaluation

5. Sterile products should be prepared at least _____ inches from the front edge of the laminar airflow hood.
   a. 6
   b. 10
   c. 2
   d. 3

6. If you add 4.5 ml of diluent to a 1.5-g vial for a final concentration of 250 mg/ml, what is the total volume in the vial after reconstitution?
   a. 4.5 ml
   b. 5 ml
   c. 5.5 ml
   d. 6 ml

7. A policies and procedures manual may provide guidance in each of the following areas except:
   a. personal orientation, training, and evaluation
   b. correct aseptic (sterile) technique
   c. activities of technicians outside the workplace
   d. position or job descriptions

8. All of the following are required on a prescription label except:
   a. name and address of the pharmacy
   b. name of the prescriber
   c. serial number of the prescription
   d. telephone number of the patient

9. A prescription can only be refilled:
   a. one time
   b. as many times as the pharmacist deems necessary
   c. as many times as the prescriber indicates on the prescription within a specified time period
   d. only at the location where it was originally filled

10. Which of the following best describes controlled substances in Schedule I?
    a. drugs with no accepted medical use in the United States
    b. drugs with a low to moderate potential for physical dependence
    c. drugs with no potential for abuse
    d. drugs available without a prescription

11. A 500-mL quantity of D10W contains how many grams of dextrose?
    a. 100 g
    b. 10 g
    c. 50 g
    d. 20 g

12. What would the check digit be for the following DEA number? AB369145_
    a. 3
    b. 8
    c. 4
    d. 0

13. The Poison Prevention Packaging Act of 1970 mandated all of the following except:
    a. Prescription drugs may be exempt if the prescriber or consumer requests noncompliant packaging.

    b. Household cleaners must be packaged in childproof containers.
    c. A limited number of prescription drugs are exempt (such as sublingual nitroglycerin).
    d. The special packaging requirements are extended to nonprescription drugs.

14. Sublingual tablets are
    a. placed under the tongue
    b. dissolved in a liquid and release bubbles
    c. placed inside the cheek
    d. chewed before swallowing

15. Which of the following IV solutions is considered isotonic?
    a. D5 ½ NS
    b. Sodium chloride 3%
    c. D10W
    d. NS

16. The Omnibus Budget Reconciliation Act of 1990 (OBRA 90) requires pharmacists to perform the following functions for patients receiving Medicaid:
    a. drug therapy review
    b. counseling
    c. financial consultation
    d. both a and b

17. The generic name for Xanax is
    a. acyclovir
    b. allopurinol
    c. alprazolam
    d. aminodarone

18. Which statement concerning Synthroid is correct?
    a. The drug strength is measured in micrograms.
    b. The usual dose is 50–100 g/day
    c. The drug is given 3 times a day.
    d. It is used to treat diabetes.

19. Prescription drugs are also known as:
    a. legend drugs
    b. new drugs
    c. over-the-counter drugs
    d. investigational drugs

20. All of the following are true concerning patient participation in an investigational drug study except:
    a. The patient must sign an informed consent.
    b. Participation is voluntary.
    c. The patient may withdraw from the study at any time.
    d. The patient must be paid.

21. You receive a prescription for Ceclor suspension 125 mg/5 mL, 1.5 tsp TID × 10 days. The correct quantity to dispense is
    a. 125 mL
    b. 150 mL with one refill
    c. 200 mL
    d. 225 mL

22. When filling a prescription for Tylenol with codeine 30 mg, a technician should do all the following except:
    a. file the prescription as a Schedule III controlled substance
    b. affix an auxiliary label cautioning against performing tasks requiring alertness or driving
    c. verify that the patient is not allergic to Tylenol or codeine
    d. inform the patient that this medication is a potent anti-inflammatory agent

23. Rx: Cortisporin gtts, use ud. Upon receiving the prescription, the technician should:
    a. fill the prescription with generic ophthalmic drops
    b. tell the patient that the prescriber must be contacted to verify ROA
    c. affix a "For the eye" auxiliary label to the container
    d. tell the patient to wash hands before administering so the drops will remain sterile

24. Which of the following drugs are commonly used to treat ulcers?
    a. digoxin and captopril
    b. prednisone and dexamethasone
    c. quinidine and quinine
    d. Tagamet and Zantac

25. Rx: Ceftriaxone 750 mg IVPB q12h. The home care technician needs to prepare a 7-day supply. How many 1-g vials will be needed?
    a. 15
    b. 6
    c. 10
    d. 11

26. What is the powder volume if a vial's final volume is 50 ml after adding 34.6 ml of diluent?
    a. 34.6 ml
    b. 15.6 ml
    c. 50 ml
    d. 15.4 ml

27. How many grams of active ingredient are in 16 oz of a 25% solution?
    a. 4
    b. 5.2
    c. 25
    d. 120

28. A computer insurance error message, "Patient not found" or "Invalid ID number," indicates that:
    a. the patient must pay cash.
    b. the patient does not appear to be enrolled in the insurance program; check for errors such as misspelling of the patient's name
    c. the patient does not have any condition that requires treatment
    d. the pharmacy must return the prescription to the patient

29. Of the following insulins, which could be added to an IV infusion?
    a. Novolog Mix 50/50
    b. Humulin NPH
    c. Humulin R
    d. Humulin 70/30

30. The portion of the prescription costs that the patient must pay in a given time period before the third-party insurer will begin paying is called a:
    a. fee-for-service
    b. co-payment
    c. deductible
    d. co-insurance

31. If a pediatric patient is to receive ampicillin oral suspension, which of the following is not necessary?
    a. Ensure that the patient is not allergic to PCN.
    b. Affix an expiration date to the label after reconstitution.
    c. Affix a "Shake well before using" label.
    d. Use aseptic technique to reconstitute the medication.

32. Which of the following resources could not be used to determine whether a parenteral medication must be filtered?
    a. the package insert
    b. *Handbook on Injectable Drugs*
    c. the IV pharmacist
    d. *American Drug Index*

33. The offer to counsel under OBRA 90 may be made:
    a. in writing
    b. orally
    c. by a technician
    d. all of the above

34. When filling an inpatient's medication drawer, the technician notices that the fill list contains both enalapril and lisinopril. The technician should:
    a. fill only one drug
    b. notify the pharmacist
    c. call the doctor
    d. tell the nurse to give the medications at least four hours apart

35. If you believe someone has presented a fraudulent prescription at your pharmacy, the appropriate action is to:
    a. discreetly call the police
    b. discreetly call the prescriber
    c. discreetly notify the pharmacist
    d. discreetly ask the customer how he got the prescription

36. You receive an order for etoposide. In preparing this drug, you should not:
    a. wear protective apparel
    b. dispose of extra drug according to policy
    c. prepare it in a biological safety cabinet
    d. prepare the drug in a horizontal laminar flow hood

37. While a mother is waiting for her child's antibiotic prescription, she asks the technician what to give the child for fever. The technician should:
    a. suggest aspirin; it's the least expensive antipyretic
    b. inform the pharmacist that the mother would like help choosing a nonprescription product
    c. offer to sell the mother acetaminophen
    d. suggest over-the-counter diphenhydramine

38. Rx: Vanceril (beclomethasone) inhaler; dispense #1; Sig: ii puffs inhaled bid. In filling the prescription, the technician should:
    a. inform the patient that this drug is a corticosteroid that has many serious side effects
    b. include the following specific directions on the label: "Inhale 2 puffs into each nostril three times a day"
    c. provide the patient the package insert included with the inhaler
    d. tell the patient to use this inhaler only when he really needs it

39. When accepting a prescription for warfarin from a patient, the technician should:
    a. notify the pharmacist if the patient is also buying aspirin; there is an interaction with these medications
    b. tell the patient to take the warfarin in the morning and the aspirin in the afternoon
    c. tell the patient to take an iron supplement because this drug thins the blood
    d. tell the patient to eat foods that are high in vitamin K

40. When selling an over-the-counter nasal decongestant spray (phenylephrine), which question can the technician answer without referring the customer to the pharmacist?
    a. Can I take this drug with my blood pressure medicine?
    b. I keep using this spray, but my nose seems to get stuffier. Should I use it more often?
    c. Is a less expensive generic available?
    d. I've had this cold for four weeks. Do you think I should see the doctor?

41. Rx: Amoxicillin suspension 5 mL po tid × 10 days. Upon review, you realize that the prescriber did not indicate the drug concentration. You should:
    a. dispense the capsules instead
    b. alert the pharmacist to the problem
    c. ask the patient which concentration he prefers
    d. prepare the prescription with the 250-mg/ml concentration because it is most frequently ordered

42. Which of the following could contribute to a medication error?
    a. failure to rotate stock appropriately
    b. preparing more than one prescription at a time
    c. not reading the drug product label carefully
    d. all the above

43. The risk of a decimal point error is reduced by writing "seven milligrams" as:
    a. 0.7 g
    b. 7 mg
    c. 7.0 mg
    d. 0.70 g

44. Which of the following drugs is stored in the pharmacy refrigerator?
    a. nystatin vaginal tablets
    b. Viroptic ophthalmic drops
    c. tetanus toxoid vaccine
    d. all the above

45. A patient calls the pharmacy asking why his heart medication is white instead of the usual yellow color. Upon investigation, it is discovered that the prescription was filled with digoxin 0.25 mg instead of the 0.125-mg strength. Which of the following is the most appropriate action to take?
    a. Tell the patient to cut the tablets in half and take one-half tablet daily.
    b. Ask the patient to bring the prescription back to the pharmacy so that you can secretly exchange it for the correct dose.
    c. Explain the situation to the pharmacist, correct the error, and document the error per procedures.
    d. Prepare a new prescription with the 0.125-mg strength and inform the patient that pharmacists are solely responsible for the accuracy of prescriptions.

46. Which of the following is not ordered on DEA Form 222?
    a. morphine
    b. hydromorphone
    c. diazepam
    d. secobarbital

47. Which of the following is not required on a unit-dose prepackaged label?
    a. drug strength
    b. lot number
    c. patient room number
    d. expiration date

48. A technician reading a medication order for a patient notices an abbreviation with which he is not familiar. Which of the following is not an acceptable way to clarify the meaning of the abbreviation?
    a. Call the prescriber.
    b. Ask the pharmacist.
    c. Refer to the lists of approved abbreviations in the policy and procedures manual.
    d. Ask the senior technician.

49. A physician calls the pharmacy asking about the maximum dose of a new medication. The technician answering the phone remembers hearing the pharmacist answer this question earlier that same day. How should the technician handle this call?
    a. Inform the physician that the maximum dose is 500 mg twice daily, because that was the dose the pharmacist gave earlier that day.
    b. Ask another technician and relay the information to the physician.
    c. Look up the answer to the question in *Facts and Comparisons* and inform the physician.
    d. Refer the question to the pharmacist.

50. A prescription with the directions to be given o.u. should be administered to:
    a. both eyes
    b. the left eye
    c. the right ear
    d. the left ear

51. The usual dose of milk of magnesia is 30 cc. This is equivalent to:
    a. 3 Tbsp
    b. 3 tsp
    c. 1 tsp
    d. 2 Tbsp

52. Which vaccine has to be stored frozen before use?
    a. oral polio
    b. injectable polio
    c. influenza
    d. pneumococcal

53. If a product is labeled to expire 8/12, what is the last date it should be used by?
    a. 8/01/12
    b. 9/01/12
    c. 7/31/12
    d. 8/31/12

54. A patient's dose of NPH U-100 insulin is 35 units qam. How much should be drawn up and administered by the nurse each morning?
    a. 0.035 ml
    b. 0.35 ml
    c. 3.5 ml
    d. 35 ml

55. Which agent is not used for the treatment of tuberculosis?
    a. pyrazinamide
    b. rifampin
    c. ethambutol
    d. vinblastine

56. Federal refill limitations for a Schedule III controlled-substance prescription are
    a. maximum of five refills and within the six-month period after initial filling of the prescription
    b. maximum of five refills and not more than one year after date of issuance
    c. maximum of ten refills and within six months of the date the prescription was written
    d. maximum of five refills and within six months of the date the prescription was written

57. Which cytotoxic drug does not require refrigeration?
    a. vinblastine
    b. cyclophosphamide
    c. asparaginase
    d. carmustine

58. The set of procedures for preparation of sterile products that is designed to prevent contamination is called:
    a. eutectic mixing
    b. filtration
    c. trituration
    d. aseptic technique

59. An example of a drug used as an anticonvulsant is
    a. aspirin
    b. chlorpromazine
    c. carbamazepined
    d. lithium

60. Which of the following statements about quality is true?
    a. Quality control is a process of checks and balances.
    b. Quality is defined by what our customers perceive.
    c. Quality improvement is an important part of meeting regulatory agency (such as JCAHO) requirements.
    d. all of the above

61. Triazolam is most commonly ordered:
    a. TID prn
    b. BID
    c. QAM
    d. QHS prn

62. Rx: Cortisporin solution ii gtts a.u. Which of the following medications should be dispensed?
    a. otic solution
    b. ophthalmic solution
    c. topical ointment
    d. ophthalmic ointment

63. Order: D5 ½ NS 2L over 10 hours. What is the IV rate?
    a. 80 ml/hr
    b. 100 ml/hr
    c. 125 ml/hr
    d. 200 ml/hr

64. Convert 1:1000 to a percent strength.
    a. 0.001%
    b. 0.01%
    c. 0.1%
    d. 1%

65. Rx: Ovral 28 i tab po daily. Disp: 3 month supply with 3 refills. If the patient's insurance pays for only a one-month supply, the technician should fill a one-month supply and adjust the refills to:
    a. 4
    b. 11
    c. 12
    d. the refills must remain at 3

66. If a patient is noted to have experienced an allergic reaction to a medication, the technician should:
    a. tell the patient that the doctor made a mistake, and refuse to fill the prescription
    b. tell the patient to take the medication anyway, since it is a doctor's order
    c. ask the patient the type of allergic reaction experienced, note the patient's response, and alert the pharmacist
    d. call the prescriber for a new prescription

67. If a prescription is written for a trade drug and is marked (according to state law) that a substitution is not allowed:
    a. a generic drug can still be dispensed if the trade is not available
    b. the specific brand-name drug must be dispensed
    c. send the patient back to the physician's office for clarification
    d. fill with a generic drug but notate that it has been substituted for the brand

68. 360 ml = _____ tablespoons
    a. 6
    b. 12
    c. 24
    d. 36

69. Three fluid ounces is equal to _____ mL.
    a. 120
    b. 90
    c. 100
    d. 150

70. Fentanyl has a concentration of 0.5 mg/mL. How many milliliters do you need for a 950-µm dose?
    a. 190 mL
    b. 0.19 mL
    c. 19 mL
    d. 1.9 mL

71. According to most insurance coverage, if a prescription is written for a brand-name product and "may substitute" is marked on it:
    a. the brand-name drug must be dispensed
    b. the generic drug must be dispensed
    c. the generic drug can be dispensed if the patient and the pharmacist agree
    d. the prescription is written incorrectly

72. The last step in processing a new prescription is
    a. computer data entry
    b. prescription filling
    c. dispensing
    d. counseling by a pharmacist

73. During prescription computer entry, the technician is responsible for all the following except:
    a. entering accurate patient demographic information
    b. entering any allergies the patient reports
    c. handling insurance claims messaging
    d. handling drug interaction messaging

74. Rx: Metronidazole 500 mg po qid × 7 days. How many 0.25-g tablets are needed to fill the prescription?
    a. 14
    b. 28
    c. 42
    d. 56

75. Rx: Penicillin 125 mg/5 ml oral susp, 250 mg po TID × 10 days. How many milliliters will be dispensed?
    a. 300 mL
    b. 150 mL
    c. 100 mL
    d. 120 mL

76. When receiving a drug–drug, drug–disease state, or drug–allergy interaction computer message, the technician should:
    a. inform the patient that the prescription cannot be filled
    b. alert the doctor to the mistake
    c. ignore the message if the patient has previously had the prescription filled
    d. alert the pharmacist to the problem

77. All of the following drugs are antidotes except:
    a. activated charcoal
    b. Digibind
    c. cefazolin
    d. naloxone

78. Which of the following is not required on a prescription label?
    a. the prescription number
    b. directions on how to take the medication
    c. the prescribing physician's name
    d. the physician's DEA number

79. The sterile parts of a syringe that may never be touched are the:
    a. plunger and barrel
    b. tip and plunger
    c. barrel and hub
    d. tip and hub

80. Why are vertical laminar airflow hoods required when preparing chemotherapy medication?
    a. They provide optimal preparer protection.
    b. Contaminated air is not blown toward the preparer.
    c. Vertical airflow hoods are not required when mixing chemotherapy drugs.
    d. both a and b

81. Which of the following medications must be protected from light?
    a. amphotericin B
    b. heparin
    c. tobramycin
    d. lanoxin

82. All of the following medications must be stored in the refrigerator, but must not be frozen, except:
    a. tetanus toxoid
    b. insulin

c. tobramycin
d. amoxicillin

83. Which of the following conditions is not commonly treated in the home care environment?
    a. sepsis
    b. osteomyelitis
    c. chronic pain
    d. malnutrition

84. All of the following medications must be prepared in a vertical laminar airflow hood except:
    a. cisplatin
    b. cyclophosphamide
    c. cefotaxime
    d. etoposide

85. All of the following drugs are laxatives except:
    a. bisacodyl tablets
    b. Citrucel powder
    c. FiberCon tablets
    d. Pancrease capsules

86. Which of the following drugs is available as an injection, topical cream, and ophthalmic solution?
    a. tobramycin
    b. furosemide
    c. gentamicin
    d. nystatin

87. Which of the following drugs is not available in an oral form and an injectable form?
    a. ranitidine
    b. furosemide
    c. prochlorperazine
    d. ibuprofen

88. Order: Tobramycin 130 mg IVPB in 100 ml of NS. How many milliliters of tobramycin 80 mg/2 ml are needed for each dose?
    a. 0.325 mL
    b. 3.25 mL
    c. 1.625 mL
    d. 1.7 mL

89. A 1000-mL bag of D5W is to infuse over 8 hr using an IV set with a drop factor of 10 gtt/ml. What is the flow rate in gtt/min?
    a. 12.5 gtt/min
    b. 21 gtt/min
    c. 22 gtt/min
    d. 125 gtt/min

90. Federal law allows _____ refills of Schedule II narcotic prescriptions.
    a. 6
    b. 1
    c. 0
    d. 12

chapter 11

Practice Certification Exam IV

This practice exam has been designed to simulate the certification exam in both the number and style of questions as well as the content. You should be able to complete this exam within two hours.

1. Which of the following drugs is indicated for the treatment of cold sores?
    a. Valtrex
    b. Zovirax
    c. Atarax
    d. Soriatane

2. The purpose of clinical pharmacy is to:
    a. dispense medications
    b. compound medication
    c. report adverse reactions or interactions to medications
    d. provide information about medication

3. Licensing and general professional oversight of pharmacists and pharmacies is carried out by:
    a. colleges of pharmacy
    b. American Pharmaceutical Society
    c. ASHP
    d. state pharmacy boards

4. A biochemically reactive component in a drug is known as:
    a. an inactive ingredient
    b. an inert ingredient
    c. a diluent
    d. an active ingredient

5. Examples of dispersions include:
    a. syrups and elixirs
    b. tinctures, fluid extracts
    c. aromatic waters, diluted acids
    d. suspensions, emulsions

6. What is the maximum number of products that can be ordered on a DEA Form 222?
    a. 1
    b. 5
    c. 8
    d. 10

7. In addition to the dosage form, the term *delivery system* refers to:
   a. use of the drug as a therapeutic, pharmacodynamic, diagnostic, prophylactic, or destructive agent
   b. the chemical composition of the drug
   c. restrictions placed on the ordering, storage, and dispensing of the drug because of its classification
   d. physical characteristics of the dosage form that determine the method of administration and the site of action of the drug

8. A customer comes into your retail pharmacy with a prescription, and his address has changed. As a technician, you should:
   a. let the pharmacist handle the situation
   b. input him into the computer system as a new patient and create a new profile
   c. update his patient profile with the new information
   d. ignore the information, because the address is not needed to fill the prescription

9. If a pharmacy technician discovers that a medication has expired, he or she should:
   a. dispense the drug if it expired within the last week
   b. discard the drug
   c. follow the pharmacy return policies
   d. dispense the drug at a discount price

10. The best source of information on compounding a medication is
    a. *Remington's Pharmaceutical Sciences*
    b. *Facts and Comparisons*
    c. *Pharmaceutical Dosage Forms and Drug Delivery Systems*
    d. *Approved Drug Products with Therapeutic Equivalence Evaluation*

11. The willingness of a patient to take a drug in the amount prescribed is called:
    a. ease of administration
    b. route of administration
    c. dosage
    d. compliance

12. Which of the following is not one of the five rights of medication administration?
    a. right route
    b. right dose
    c. right medication
    d. right doctor

13. Good Manufacturing Practices are regulated by the:
    a. Texas State Board of Pharmacy
    b. FDA
    c. DEA
    d. Manufacturers of America

14. Which of the following would most likely not be found in a pharmacy policy and procedures manual?
    a. hiring practices
    b. management of dangerous drugs
    c. inventory control of pharmaceuticals
    d. good compounding practices

15. How many milliliters of a 250-mg/5-ml liquid are needed for a 0.75-g dose?
    a. 1.5 ml
    b. 7.5 ml
    c. 10 ml
    d. 15 ml

16. A person with a thiamine deficiency has an inadequate supply of:
    a. vitamin B-12
    b. vitamin B-6
    c. vitamin D
    d. vitamin B-1

17. A 500-mg/250-ml dopamine IV is infusing at 1000 mcg per minute. What is the flow rate in ml/hr?
    a. 10 ml/hr
    b. 20 ml/hr
    c. 30 ml/hr
    d. 50 ml/hr

18. Which of the following is not a factor that affects how a prescriber doses a medication?
    a. weight
    b. insurance
    c. age
    d. physical condition

19. Which of the following dosage forms deteriorates and loses potency faster than tablets?
    a. suppositories
    b. oral inhalers
    c. liquids
    d. capsules

20. Repackaging large, non–patient-specific quantities of medications to be used over long periods of time is an example of _____ repackaging.
    a. extemporaneous
    b. batch
    c. patient-specific
    d. unit dose

21. How much 70% sorbitol is needed to prepare 8 fluid ounces of 50% sorbitol?
    a. 5.7 ml
    b. 11.2 ml
    c. 171.4 ml
    d. 336 ml

22. Which of the following topical medications requires special chemotherapy handling?
    a. Hytone 2.5%
    b. Kenalog 2.5%
    c. Efudex 5%
    d. Elidel 1%

23. Using the drug's _____ is the best method for pharmacy technicians to ensure that they are dispensing the correct drug.
    a. expiration date
    b. lot number
    c. wholesaler item number
    d. NDC

24. Pharmacies are required to have which of the following types of pharmacy balance?
    a. electronic
    b. Class A
    c. Class B
    d. Harvard Trip

25. Of the following equipment, which would least likely be used to compound a prescription for an oral suspension?
    a. mortar
    b. compounding slab
    c. graduated cylinder
    d. pestle

26. You receive a rejected insurance claim stating "refill too early." Which of the following could be the potential reason for the rejected claim?
    a. wrong patient code
    b. wrong quantity dispensed
    c. wrong days' supply
    d. patient does not have current coverage

27. A PRN medication is one that is
    a. given continuously around the clock
    b. given at set time intervals
    c. given only in response to a specific parameter
    d. given rectally

28. Which of the following medications is contraindicated in pregnant women?
    a. indomethacin
    b. isotretinoin
    c. ibuprofen
    d. itraconazole

29. Which of the following equipment is used to compound TPNs?
    a. Pyxis
    b. ScriptPro
    c. Automix
    d. Omnicell

30. Which of the following is indicated for active duodenal ulcers?
    a. Ropinirole HCl
    b. Risperidone
    c. Risedronate Sodium
    d. Ranitidine

31. A patient asks what OTC medication she should take for persistent heartburn. The pharmacy technician should:
    a. tell the patient to take Prilosec OTC
    b. tell the patient to talk to her doctor
    c. tell the patient to talk with the pharmacist on duty
    d. tell the patient to go to the emergency room

32. Aluminum hydroxide and diphenhydramine are mixed in a 3:1 ratio. How much of each is required to make 4 oz of suspension?
    a. 100 ml/20 ml
    b. 90 ml/30 ml
    c. 75 ml/25 ml
    d. 60 ml/60 ml

33. Rx: Platinol IV 20 mg/m^2/day for 5 days. If the patient's BSA is 1.52 m^2, how much of the drug must be drawn up for one dose if the concentration of the Platinol vial is 50 mg/50 ml.
    a. 20 ml
    b. 30 ml
    c. 30.4 ml
    d. 50 ml

34. Rx: Lasix 40 mg IV q8h. How many 10-ml furosemide, 10-mg/ml multidose vials should the pharmacy technician send for a 24-hr supply?
    a. 1
    b. 2
    c. 3
    d. 4

35. What is the IV rate (ml/hr) if the patient has 2000 ml of D5W infused every 24 hr?
    a. 38 ml/hr
    b. 48 ml/hr
    c. 83 ml/hr
    d. 84 ml/hr

36. Penicillin suspension is available in a concentration of 250 mg/5 ml. How many teaspoons are required for a 375-mg dose?
    a. ½ tsp
    b. ¾ tsp
    c. 1½ tsp
    d. 1¾ tsp

37. The drug rifampin requires which of the following auxiliary labels?
    a. take with food or milk
    b. may cause discoloration of urine or feces
    c. do not take with aspirin
    d. may cause photosensitivity

38. A 10-ml U-100 insulin vial has a concentration of:
    a. 100 units per 10 ml
    b. 100 units per ml
    c. 100 units per 0.5 ml
    d. 100 units per 100 ml

39. A patient who is currently taking warfarin should not take which of the following controlled-substance medications?
    a. meperidine
    b. Percocet
    c. Dilaudid
    d. Percodan

40. Which of the following drugs would most likely have an "automatic stop order" in a hospital pharmacy?
    a. antitussives
    b. IV infusions
    c. investigational drugs
    d. antibiotics

41. Convert 1:10,000 to a percent strength.
    a. 0.0001%
    b. 0.001%
    c. 0.01%
    d. 0.1%

42. Pharmacy technicians deliver medications to nursing stations and pick up new physician's orders during their:
    a. IV delivery rounds
    b. chemotherapy delivery rounds
    c. floorstock delivery rounds
    d. medication delivery rounds

43. Which of the following routes of administration has the quickest onset of action?
    a. IV
    b. ID
    c. po
    d. pr

44. Of the following information, which is not required on a unit-dose package?
    a. expiration date
    b. patient name
    c. lot number
    d. drug strength

45. The PPI for an oral inhaler prescription is required to be dispensed:
    a. only the first time the prescription is dispensed
    b. once a year
    c. each time the prescription is dispensed
    d. only upon the prescriber's request

46. What is the cost for 60 tablets if the pharmacy's cost is $42.10 per 100 tabs and a 25% markup is applied?
    a. $25.26
    b. $30.31
    c. $52.63
    d. $31.58

47. Which of the following medications is indicated for congestive heart failure?
    a. phenytoin
    b. glyburide
    c. valacyclovir
    d. captopril

48. How many grams of hydrocortisone is in 120 grams of hydrocortisone 0.5% ointment?
    a. 0.6 grams
    b. 6 grams
    c. 60 grams
    d. 66 grams

49. The concentration of an injectable drug is 30 mg/5 ml. What volume is required for a 38.4-mg dose?
    a. 5.6 ml
    b. 6.4 ml
    c. 7.7 ml
    d. 7.8 ml

50. The recommended dose for cefadroxil is 30 mg/kg/day in two divided doses. How much should be given in each dose for a child who weighs 40 lb?
    a. 1200 mg
    b. 600 mg
    c. 545 mg
    d. 273 mg

51. How many 125-mg doses are in 10 g of drug?
    a. 10 doses
    b. 20 doses
    c. 40 doses
    d. 80 doses

52. The term *gauge* refers to:
    a. the diameter of the needle's shaft
    b. the length of the needed
    c. the size of the needle's lumen
    d. the needle's bevel

53. If the pharmacy technician receives an insurance error message stating an invalid "IDC-9" code, this means that what information is incorrect?
    a. drug strength
    b. drug manufacturer
    c. drug NDC
    d. patient diagnosis

54. Rx: Piroxicam 20 mg ii po bid. How many milligrams will the patient take in a 24-hr period?
    a. 20 mg
    b. 40 mg
    c. 80 mg
    d. 120 mg

55. How many 10-mg morphine tablets are needed to prepare 100 ml of a 1-mg/ml morphine solution?
    a. 1 tablet
    b. 5 tablets
    c. 10 tablets
    d. 20 tablets

56. A chemotherapy spill kit is required to be in close proximity of the preparer when an IV of which of the following drugs is compounded?
    a. famciclovir
    b. acyclovir
    c. cyclophosphamide
    d. morphine sulfate

57. The trade name for oseltamivir phosphate is
    a. Tenormin
    b. Temovate
    c. Theo-dur
    d. Tamiflu

58. Which of the following sublingual drugs must be dispensed in its original glass container?
    a. isosorbide
    b. nitroglycerin
    c. zolpidem
    d. lorazepam

59. If 30 grams of ointment contain 250 mg of drug, what is the percent strength of the preparation?
    a. 0.1%
    b. 0.38%
    c. 0.48%
    d. 0.83%

60. If a prescriber discontinues a patient's investigational drug, what should the pharmacy do with the remaining drug?
    a. return it to the physician
    b. return it to the patient
    c. destroy the investigational drug
    d. return the drug to the manufacturer

61. If the pharmacy inventory is shelved alphabetically by generic name, under which letter would the drug Pamelor be found?
    a. B
    b. D
    c. N
    d. P

62. To maintain perpetual inventory control, the pharmacy must update records:
    a. whenever inventory is purchased or sold
    b. whenever sales figures are updated
    c. to identify low turnover
    d. to generate orders

63. 0023-022-11. The bolded portion of the NDC identifies the:
    a. drug strength
    b. manufacturer
    c. drug product
    d. package size

64. What is meant by the term *drug inventory rotation*?
    a. Using the drugs with the longest expiration date first
    b. Making sure that drugs with the longest expiration date are placed at the front of the shelf
    c. Making sure that drugs with the shortest expiration date are placed at the front of the shelf
    d. Making sure that drugs with the shortest expiration date are placed at the back of the shelf

65. The purpose of a hospital formulary is to:
    a. provide a listing of drugs approved by the insurance company
    b. provide a listing of the institution's approved drug products
    c. provide a listing of all FDA-approved drugs available
    d. provide the pharmacy technician with a listing of drugs in the pharmacy inventory

66. Tylenol #3 is listed on which schedule of controlled substances?
    a. Schedule I
    b. Schedule II
    c. Schedule III
    d. Schedule IV

67. Which of the following pharmacy records is most likely to be used to track medication that has been recalled?
    a. productivity report
    b. drug utilization report
    c. temperature logs
    d. purchase orders

68. The term *inventory turnover rate* refers to:
    a. the delivery turnaround time from the wholesaler
    b. how often the pharmacy rotates stock
    c. how often the pharmacy uses inventory
    d. how the inventory is ordered

69. The expiration date on a medication bottle states 7/12. When does the medication expire?
    a. July 1, 2012
    b. June 1, 2012
    c. July 31, 2012
    d. July 31, 2013

70. Which of the following drugs must be ordered using DEA Form 222?
    a. diazepam
    b. acetaminophen with codeine tablets
    c. meperidine
    d. guiafenesin with codeine liquid

71. Which of the following medications is indicated for the treatment of diabetes?
    a. Actonel
    b. Actos
    c. Adderall
    d. Advair

72. The term *inventory PAR level* refers to:
    a. the maximum quantity of inventory to be kept on the shelves
    b. the minimum quantity of inventory to be kept on the shelves
    c. the quantity of drug that should be ordered each time
    d. both a and c

73. Which of the following reference sources supplies the same information as is on a package insert?
    a. Red Book
    b. Orange Book
    c. PDR
    d. *Drug Facts and Comparisons*

74. Which of the following is indicated for the treatment of depression?
    a. Patanol
    b. Paxil
    c. Pepcid
    d. Peridex

75. A maintenance medication is not in stock. What is the proper procedure for the technician to follow?
    a. tell the patient he has no choice but to go to a different pharmacy
    b. tell the patient that the prescription cannot be filled
    c. inform the pharmacist and see if she can call the prescriber and ask to substitute a drug that is in stock
    d. ask the patient if you can call an alternate pharmacy of his choice to see if that pharmacy stocks the medication

76. Which of the following would not result if a pharmacy technician filed an inaccurate insurance claim for a prescription?
    a. denied claim
    b. delayed claim
    c. increase in insurance payment to the pharmacy
    d. decrease in insurance payment to the pharmacy

77. A drug product that requires refrigeration should be stored at a temperature between:
    a. −25 –and −10°C
    b. 2 and 8°C
    c. 8 and 15°C
    d. 20 and 25°C

78. When there is an incorrect box count, the technician receiving the order should:
    a. not accept any part of the order
    b. accept the order as complete
    c. document the incorrect box count with the delivery person
    d. accept the order and hope the wholesaler sends the balance

79. Which class of recalls can cause severe adverse effects or death?
    a. Class I
    b. Class II
    c. Class III
    d. Class IV

80. Material Safety Data Sheets are required by which of the following?
    a. FDA
    b. HIPAA
    c. USP
    d. OSHA

81. Which of the following drugs is NOT exempt from the Poison Prevention Packaging Act?
    a. oral inhalers
    b. nitroglycerin sl tablets
    c. unit-dose medications used in an institutional setting
    d. diazepam

82. If the refill section is left blank, the pharmacy can:
    a. give the patient as many refills as he wants
    b. assume that no refills were intended to be given
    c. give the patient a 1-year supply
    d. not fill the prescription

83. Which of the following laws requires pharmacists to counsel Medicaid patients?
    a. HIPAA
    b. OSHA
    c. OBRA 90
    d. COBRA

84. When ordering schedule II controlled substances, who signs the order form?
    a. the narcotic technician
    b. the pharmacist on duty
    c. the pharmacy manager
    d. the pharmacy person with power of attorney

85. Compounding equipment used in the IV room must be cleaned at least:
    a. once a week
    b. once a day
    c. once an hour
    d. once a year

86. How often should pharmaceutical balances and scales be professionally certified for accuracy?
    a. once a month
    b. every 6 months
    c. every year
    d. every 10 years

87. Which of the following is considered a covered entity under HIPAA regulations?
    a. health care provider
    b. health plan
    c. health care clearinghouse
    d. all the above

88. Which of the following technologies is only used in a retail or outpatient pharmacy setting?
    a. Pyxis
    b. Omnicell
    c. ScriptPro
    d. AcuDose Rx

89. Where can a technician find information on the pharmacy's best practices for quality drug delivery?
    a. HIPAA notice of disclosure
    b. MSDS book
    c. JCAHO website
    d. P&P manual

90. Which of the following would pay for a person's outpatient expenses?
    a. Medicare Part A
    b. Medicare Part B
    c. Medicare Part C
    d. Medicare Part D

Practice Certification Exam V

This practice exam has been designed to simulate the certification exam in both the number and style of questions as well as the content. You should be able to complete this exam within two hours.

1. The portion of the cost of a prescription that a patient with third-party insurance must pay is the:
   a. co-payment
   b. deductible
   c. U&C
   d. MAC

2. All of the following define the term *drug* except:
   a. an article intended for use in the diagnosis, cure, mitigation, treatment, or prevention of disease in humans or other animals
   b. an article recognized in the USP, the NF, and the Homeopathic Pharmacopoeia of the United States
   c. a device used for a life-sustaining or life-supporting function
   d. an article (other than food) intended to affect the structure or any function of the body

3. All of the following methods for filing prescriptions are allowed except:
   a. a system using three prescription file drawers: one drawer for CII prescriptions, one drawer for CIII, CIV, and CV prescriptions, and one drawer for all others
   b. a system using two prescription file drawers: one drawer for all controlled-substance prescriptions and one drawer for all other prescriptions
   c. a system using five prescription file drawers: one drawer for CII, one drawer for CIII, one drawer for CIV, one drawer for CV, and one drawer for all other prescriptions.
   d. a system using two prescription file drawers: one drawer for CII prescriptions and one drawer for all other prescriptions including CIII, CIV, and CV

4. Each of the following is a characteristic desired in an intravenous solution except:
   a. pH of 6
   b. sterility
   c. clarity
   d. pyrogen-free

5. How many 5-mg tablets are needed to fill the following prescription? Prednisone 5-mg tablets per sliding scale, 20 mg daily × 2 d, 15 mg daily × 2 d, 5 mg bid × 2 d, 2.5 mg bid × 2 d, 2.5 mg daily × 2 d
   a. 20 tabs
   b. 21 tabs
   c. 22 tabs
   d. 15 tabs

6. Calculate the flow rate for an IV of 1000 mL to run over 8 hr with a set calibrated at 20 gtt/mL.
   a. 42 gtt/min
   b. 17 gtt/min
   c. 125 gtt/min
   d. 50 gtt/min

7. Which of the following information is not required to be on a retail prescription label?
   a. pharmacy name and phone number
   b. prescription number
   c. patient's phone number
   d. prescriber's name

8. An air vent on a vented administration set should be a _____-micron filter vent to be considered a sterilizing filter.
   a. 0.2
   b. 0.5
   c. 5
   d. 10

9. How long will it take a 150-ml IV to infuse at a rate of 50 ml/hr?
   a. 1 hr
   b. 2 hr
   c. 2.5 hr
   d. 3 hr

10. A _____ is a device designed to reduce the risk of airborne contamination during the preparation of an IV admixture by providing an ultra-clean environment.
    a. laminar airflow hood
    b. HEPA filter
    c. autoclave
    d. automix

11. _____ is a procedure conducted under controlled conditions in a manner that minimizes the chance of contamination resulting from the introduction of microorganisms.
    a. Pharmaceutical care
    b. Aseptic technique
    c. Sterilization
    d. Autoclaving

12. Maximum and minimum inventory levels for each drug are known as:
    a. reorder points
    b. M&M inventory
    c. POS points
    d. the Maxim system

13. _____ is an unintended side effect of a medication that is negative or in some way injurious to a patient's health.
    a. A contraindication
    b. An adverse effect
    c. An indication
    d. A warning

14. The _____ is a form used in institutional settings to prescribe medications.
    a. prescription
    b. medication order
    c. MAR
    d. fill list

15. If an accident occurs involving a hazardous substance that is stored in the pharmacy, what document will provide instructions on actions that need to be taken?
    a. policies and procedure manual
    b. MSDS
    c. employee handbook
    d. OSHA "Right to Know" pamphlet

16. A pharmacy fills three prescriptions using sulfur powder. The first prescription uses 10 g, the second uses 0.5 kg, and the third uses 25 mg. What was the total amount of sulfur used to fill the three prescriptions?
    a. 510.025 g
    b. 35.5 g
    c. 510.25 g
    d. 60.25 g

17. _____ occurs when a drug is substantially degraded or destroyed by the liver's enzymes before it reaches the circulatory system.
    a. Enzyme induction
    b. Tolerance
    c. A first-pass effect
    d. Metabolism

18. The _____ classified drugs according to their potential for abuse.
    a. Comprehensive Drug Abuse Prevention and Control Act
    b. Medical Device Amendment
    c. Controlled Substances Act
    d. Anabolic Steroid Control Act

19. The abbreviation PR stands for
    a. per recommendation
    b. previous records
    c. rectally
    d. percent reduction

20. All of the following concerning DEA Form 222 are true except:
    a. It is in triplicate.
    b. Copy 1 and Copy 2 are forwarded to the supplier.
    c. Multiple items may be ordered per line.
    d. There are 10 lines on the form.

21. The _____ is a price that is determined by a survey of the usual and customary prices for a prescription within a given geographic area.
    a. MAC
    b. deductible
    c. U&C
    d. UAC

22. Administrations of large volumes of solution over several hours at a slow, constant rate are known as:
    a. intermittent infusion
    b. continuous infusion
    c. a piggyback
    d. an infusion pump

23. The DEA form used to surrender C-II medications for disposition is
    a. Form 222
    b. Form 224
    c. Form 41
    d. Form 363

24. Administration of relatively small volumes of solution over a short time at specific intervals is known as:
    a. continuous infusion
    b. TPN
    c. intermittent infusion
    d. enteral nutrition

25. Add 1.17 kg, 1.59 g, and 260 mg.
    a. 262.76 g
    b. 1461.35 g
    c. 3.02 g
    d. 1171.85 g

26. Which of the following are one-time-use containers?
    a. an ampoule
    b. an IV piggyback
    c. a unit-dose package
    d. all the above

27. Which of the following units of measure represents the smallest unit of weight?
    a. gram
    b. milligram
    c. kilogram
    d. microgram

28. The word _____ indicates directions for use.
    a. magma
    b. scribe
    c. signa
    d. indication

29. When preparing a TPN solution containing calcium, phosphate, and other ingredients, which of the following statements is true?
    a. The calcium and phosphate should be mixed together in the same syringe before being injected into the TPN solution.
    b. The calcium should be added first, then all other additives, then add the phosphate last.
    c. The phosphate should be added first, then all other additives, then add the calcium last.
    d. The calcium and phosphate should be added last, after all other additives.

30. A system that maintains a continuous record of every item in inventory so that it always shows stock on hand is known as:
    a. perpetual inventory
    b. a POS system
    c. turnover
    d. reorder points

31. A cough-and-cold tablet contains the following amounts of active ingredients:

acetaminophen	325 mg
chlorpheniramine maleate	2 mg
pseudoephedrine hydrochloride	30 mg
dextromethorphan	15 mg
guaifenesin	100 mg

    The pharmacy has 2 kg of acetaminophen, 5 g of chlorpheniramine maleate, and an unlimited supply of the other ingredients. How many tablets can be prepared?
    a. 6153
    b. 2500
    c. 2885
    d. 5000

32. Sodium chloride is _____ solution.
    a. a hypotonic
    b. an isotonic
    c. a hypertonic
    d. none of the above

33. Capsules are medications enclosed in gelatin. They are available in several sizes. Which of the following sizes is the smallest?
    a. 000
    b. 00
    c. 0
    d. 1

34. A person diagnosed with GERD is likely to be prescribed which of the following medications?
    a. propranolol
    b. ciprofloxin
    c. phenytoin
    d. esomeprazole

35. Which of the following is not true regarding nitroglycerin?
    a. It is indicated for angina pectoris.
    b. It is sensitive to light and moisture, so it should be dispensed in amber glass containers.
    c. It is an exception to the Poison Prevention Act.
    d. It is stable for one year after dispensing.

36. A bulk vial of cefazolin indicates an expiration date of May 2012. Which of the following statements is true regarding the use of this cefazolin vial?
    a. The vial may be used for up to one year after the printed expiration date.
    b. The vial must be used by May 1, 2012.
    c. The vial can be used through the last day of May 2012.
    d. The vial may be used for up to six months after the printed expiration date.

37. A patient is receiving Timentin 3.1 g q6h via a CADD Plus pump at home. Which of the following information is mandatory on a label in the home care setting?
    a. patient address
    b. prescriber's phone number
    c. drug NDC
    d. transcribed directions

38. Which controlled-substance classification includes sedative and hypnotic drugs?
    a. C II
    b. C III
    c. C IV
    d. C V

39. You receive an order to prepare 250 mg of dobutamine in a 100-mL CADD cassette with NS as the diluent. Dobutamine is available as a 12.5-mg/mL solution. How many milliliters of dobutamine do you need to prepare this prescription?

    a. 20 mL
    b. 40 mL
    c. 200 mL
    d. 400 mL

40. How much 10% dextrose can be prepared from 500 ml of 70% dextrose?
    a. 3500 ml
    b. 1400 ml
    c. 7140 ml
    d. 2050 ml

41. You are asked to make fluorouracil 4000 mg in 1000 mL of sodium chloride 0.9%. What auxiliary label should be placed on the prepared admixture?
    a. Protect from light.
    b. Caution: Federal law prohibits the transfer of this drug to any person other than the patient for whom it was prescribed.
    c. Chemotherapy/biohazard.
    d. Administer with food or milk.

42. A pharmacy technician is preparing heparin 25,000 units in 500 ml of dextrose 5% in water. The concentration on the label should read:
    a. 250 units/ml
    b. 125 units/ml
    c. 100 units/ml
    d. 50 units/ml

43. The pharmacist asks you to check the compatibility of parenteral phenytoin with sodium chloride 0.9%. Which reference should you select to find this information?
    a. *Handbook of Injectable Drugs*
    b. *Remington's Pharmaceutical Sciences*
    c. *Medication Teaching Manual: The Guide to Patient Drug Information*
    d. *Drug Facts and Comparisons*

44. In which of the following functions may a well-trained technician participate?
    a. documenting investigational drug use
    b. preparing chemotherapeutic agents
    c. purchasing and inventory control
    d. all of the above

45. Checking the temperature of a refrigerator that stores medications on a daily basis is
    a. an example of a quality-control mechanism used to meet Joint Commission requirements
    b. a method to assure proper storage of medications and avoid waste
    c. a mechanism to satisfy a technicain's job duties as set by the pharmacy director
    d. all the above

46. In a hospital pharmacy, the technician can assist the pharmacist in all the following ways except:

    a. dispensing STAT medications without the pharmacist's approval

    b. alerting the pharmacist when a medication order appears to be written in error (for example, overdose)

    c. obtaining a patient's lab results

    d. alerting the pharmacist if a nonformulary drug has been ordered

47. All of the following statements are false except:

    a. A technician needs a license to practice in a central pharmacy and a separate license to practice in a satellite pharmacy.

    b. The technician can dispense medications without a final check by a pharmacist.

    c. A technician can answer questions related to patient-specific drug information.

    d. A technician can retrieve lab data for the pharmacist to use in making clinical judgments on patient care.

48. To be considered a generic equivalent for a trade-named drug product, the substitute must be

    a. bioequivalent

    b. the same color

    c. made by the same manufacturer

    d. the same shape

49. Cleaning a vertical laminar airflow hood includes using which of the following agents?

    a. isopropyl alcohol

    b. sterile water

    c. povidone-iodine

    d. both a and b

50. Which of the following statements is (are) true regarding the technician's role in formulary issues?

    a. The technician can screen for orders that are nonformulary and alert the pharmacist.

    b. The technician can alert the purchasing agent when the par level of a formulary item is getting low.

    c. The technician can initially screen orders that are considered expensive or have potential for complication and alert the pharmacist.

    d. all of the above

51. Which of the following are ways in which the technician can participate in quality improvement?

    a. mapping out the work flow of a system or process requiring improvement

    b. collecting data for the evaluation of a process

    c. calling the physician to discuss appropriate drug therapy

    d. both a and b

52. If a patient tells you that his six-month-old child ingested "some" iron tablets, the pharmacy technician is responsible for:

    a. looking up the toxic dose of ferrous sulfate in *Facts and Comparisons*

    b. instructing the parent to buy activated charcoal

    c. telling the parent that "some" iron tablets will not harm the child

    d. instructing the parent to call the local poison control center

53. When giving drug information to the patient, which of the following is the least desirable source?

    a. patient package insert

    b. *USP DI Advice for the Patient*

    c. a manufacturer's "patient education" brochure

    d. a drug package insert

54. At cart fill, you identify an order to refill both cisapride and fluconazole for a patient. You should:

    a. notify the pharmacist of a possible drug interaction

    b. fill the cart, because a drug interaction screening has already been done by the pharmacist

    c. do nothing, because no drug interaction exists between the two agents

    d. call the physician to change the antibiotic

55. *American Drug Index* provides the following information:

    a. brand-to-generic-name cross-referencing

    b. available medication dosage forms

    c. manufacturer name, address, and phone number

    d. all of the above

56. Questions that may be answered by Material Safety Data Sheets include all of the following except:

    a. What precautions must be taken when preparing and dispensing Adriamycin?

    b. What is the dosing of activated charcoal for accidental poisoning?

    c. How should an employee exposed to Adriamycin be treated?

    d. How should a chemotherapy spill be cleaned?

57. All of the following are required when filling and dispensing a prescription for a metaproterenol oral metered-dose inhaler except:

    a. auxiliary label: For oral inhalation only

    b. auxiliary label: Shake well

    c. patient instructions

    d. auxiliary label: Take with food

58. A retail pharmacy is having a sale on an OTC drug. If the item's regular price is $6.80 and it is to be marked down 40%, what will be the selling price of the item?
    a. $2.72
    b. $4.08
    c. $4.80
    d. $2.27

59. The most common and uncomplicated route of administration is
    a. intravenous
    b. intramuscular
    c. oral
    d. sublingual

60. A troche is also known as:
    a. an effervescent tablet
    b. a lozenge
    c. a granule
    d. a gelatin capsule

61. Pastilles are
    a. placed under the tongue and dissolved
    b. inserted into the vagina
    c. placed into the pouch of the lower eyelid
    d. held in the mouth and sucked

62. Extended-release dosage forms are formulated to:
    a. have longer shelf lives than regularly formulated products
    b. release medication slowly over an extended period of time
    c. increase the number of doses a patient must take in a day
    d. lengthen the amount of time before a prescription must be refilled

63. Which of the following routes of medication administration is not a parenteral route?
    a. subq
    b. pr
    c. I.D.
    d. I.M.

64. Which of the following drugs should be stored in the hospital's CII stock?
    a. diazepam
    b. codeine with acetaminophen
    c. phenobarbital
    d. hydromorphone

65. A patient is being provided with TPN, and the following order has been sent to the pharmacy. If the pharmacy stocks magnesium sulfate 10% (0.8 mEq/ml) in a 10-mL vial, what is the volume of drug that should be added if 24 mEq/2 L is ordered?
    a. 0.3 mL
    b. 0.8 mL
    c. 2.15 mL
    d. 30 mL

66. Which of the following vitamins is needed for proper blood clotting?
    a. vitamin A
    b. vitamin D
    c. vitamin E
    d. vitamin K

67. As a pharmacy technician in a home care environment, you might be responsible for which of the following tasks?
    a. picking and packing medical supplies
    b. delivering supplies to the patient's home
    c. purchasing drugs and medical supplies
    d. all of the above

68. A type of reimbursement whereby a pharmacy receives a predetermined amount of money for a defined group of patients regardless of the number of prescriptions filled is
    a. fee-for-service
    b. co-payment
    c. capitation
    d. no payment

69. Typical data collected from the patient at the prescription take-in window include:
    a. weight for children and infants
    b. allergies
    c. emergency phone numbers
    d. all of the above

70. What volume of medication will deliver a dose of 65 mg if the vial label reads 10 mg/5 ml?
    a. 6.5 ml
    b. 13 ml
    c. 32.5 ml
    d. 130 ml

71. Examples of quality-control measures utilized when preparing an IVPB include:
    a. pulling the drug from the shelf and double-checking to ensure that the vial is correct
    b. calculating the correct dose and volume to withdraw from the vial to ensure that the vial is correct
    c. checking the IVPB for particulate matter after injecting the medication
    d. all of the above

72. The _____ is a set amount that must be paid by the patient for each benefit period before the insurer will cover additional expenses.
    a. co-payment
    b. deductible
    c. garnishment
    d. MAC

73. Personal protective equipment should be used properly when handling hazardous medications. This consists of:
    a. gloves
    b. gown
    c. mask
    d. all the above

74. How many tablets will be dispensed for a prescription indicating that a patient is to take 1 tablet po bid for 30 days?
    a. 30
    b. 60
    c. 90
    d. 120

75. Of the following tasks involved in pharmacy practice, which is allowed by law for technicians to perform?
    a. giving or receiving a verbal copy
    b. counseling a patient on the use of his medication
    c. receiving a verbal order from a physician
    d. filling a unit-dose cart

76. What organization requires that oral products be stored separate from inhaled products, topical preparations be separated from injectables, and so on?
    a. DEA
    b. PTCB
    c. APHA
    d. Joint Commission

77. An automatic stop order is most likely to be issued for which of the following meds?
    a. clonidine 0.3-mg tablets
    b. acetaminophen/codeine 325-mg/60-m tablets
    c. amlodipine 5-mg tablets
    d. furosemide 40-mg tablets

78. Which of the following is equal to 32 tbsp?
    a. 473 ml
    b. 3785 ml
    c. 16 fluid oz
    d. 480 g

79. Amphotericin B should be mixed only in _____ for compatibility.
    a. 0.9% sodium chloride
    b. LR
    c. 0.45% sodium chloride
    d. D5W

80. Which of the following is not an automated dispensing system that might found in an inpatient pharmacy?
    a. Script-Pro
    b. Omnicell
    c. Pyxis
    d. Rx Robot

81. After preparing IV doxorubicin, how should the technicians dispose of the used needles?
    a. Dispose of needles in an approved biohazard sharps container without recapping.
    b. Bend needles so they cannot possibly be reused.
    c. Dispose of needles in an approved hazardous sharps container without recapping.
    d. Discard needles into a cardboard box that has been identified for needle waste

82. Which of the following drugs is indicated for the treatment of weight management?
    a. phentermine
    b. phenobarbital
    c. phanazopyridine
    d. paroxetine

83. Of the following information, which would not be found on a prescription label?
    a. dispensing pharmacist's initials
    b. name of medication
    c. prescriber's signature
    d. patient's name

84. Which of the following would be stored within the topical section of the pharmacy's inventory?
    a. Erythromycin 2% soln
    b. Mylanta liquid
    c. Nystatin 100,000 units/ml susp
    d. Gentamicin 80-mg/2-ml inj

85. Which of the following drugs would not likely be found on an emergency crash cart?
    a. epinephrine injection
    b. cimetidine injection
    c. lidocaine injection
    d. dopamine injection

LINE #	PATIENT'S NAME	QUANTITY DISPENSED	QUANTITY RECEIVED	CURRENT BALANCE
1	Beginning Balance			87
2	Barbara Jones	42		44
3	Received from wholesaler		100	144
4	Thomas Watkins	24		120

86. On the above perpetual inventory for a Schedule II controlled substance, what line contains an error?

    a. 1
    b. 2
    c. 3
    d. 4

87. If a patient experiences an adverse reaction to a prescription, the reaction should be reported to:

    a. the Joint Commission
    b. MedWatch
    c. the state board of pharmacy
    d. the drug manufacturer

88. How many 1-liter bags of dextrose 5% will the IV technician need to send for a 24-hour supply if the infusion rate is 125 mL/hr?

    a. 6
    b. 5

    c. 4
    d. 3

89. What is the pharmacy technician's best defense against contamination when preparing patient prescriptions?

    a. spraying with Lysol
    b. proper hand washing
    c. mopping with chlorine bleach
    d. wearing gloves

90. Which of the following medications is not used to treat hypertension?

    a. lisinopril
    b. terazosin
    c. metoprolol
    d. etodolac

Math Practice Test I

Complete this test to review pharmacy calculations.

1. Rx: Diphenhydramine 0.1% solution, 500 ml. How much diphenhydramine 0.25% solution will be needed to prepare the prescription?
   a. 100 ml
   b. 200 ml
   c. 350 ml
   d. 400 ml

2. Rx: Zovirax 400-mg tabs, i po, 5× daily. Dispense: 100 tabs. What is the
   days' supply for the prescription?
   a. 10
   b. 20
   c. 30
   d. 50

3. Rx: Albuterol oral solution, 3 mg po tid. Disp: 14-day supply. If the pharmacy dispenses albuterol 2-mg/5-ml solution, how much is needed to fill
   the prescription?
   a. 7.5 ml
   b. 42 ml
   c. 126 ml
   d. 315 ml

4. Rx: Clotrimazole 0.5% ointment, 60 grams. How many grams of clotrimazole 1% should be mixed with ointment base to prepare the prescription?
   a. 5 grams
   b. 15 grams
   c. 30 grams
   d. 60 grams

5. Digoxin 0.25-mg tabs cost $10.23/100 tabs and the pharmacy applies a
   32% markup on cost plus a $4.50 dispensing fee. What will the patient be
   charged for 90 tabs?
   a. $16.65
   b. $13.71
   c. $12.15
   d. $9.21

6. How much sorbitol 70% must be mixed with sterile water to prepare 1 L of sorbitol 25% solution?

    a. 280 mL
    b. 357 mL
    c. 643 mL
    d. 720 mL

7. 4350 ml = _____ tbsp

    a. 9
    b. 145
    c. 870
    d. 290

8. How many teaspoons are in 12.5 ml?

    a. 1½
    b. 2
    c. 2¼
    d. 2½

9. Order: NS 1 L with 35,000 units of heparin infusing @ 20 ml/hr. Calculate the hourly dosage of heparin.

    a. 350 units/hr
    b. 700 units/hr
    c. 1,400 units/hr
    d. 3500 units/hr

10. Rx: Cimetidine 300-mg tab po qid- Disp: 3 month supply. How many cimetidine 300-mg tabs are needed to fill the prescription?

    a. 120
    b. 180
    c. 240
    d. 360

11. Rx: Cleocin 150-mg capsules, 300 mg po bid. Disp: 100 caps. What is the prescription's days' supply?

    a. 10
    b. 20
    c. 25
    d. 30

12. Dr. William Wiggins is treating Edna Edwards with Amoxil for an ear infection. He writes a prescription for Amoxil 30 mg/kg/day in divided doses q8h for 10 days. Edna is six months old and weighs 26.4 lb. How much will be given to Edna in each dose if the pharmacy dispenses amoxicillin 125-mg/5-ml susp?

    a. 3.75 ml
    b. 4.8 ml
    c. 5 ml
    d. 5.2 ml

13. You have a 500-ml bag of D5 ½ NS. How many grams of NaCl does this bag contain?

    a. 7.5 grams
    b. 4.5 grams
    c. 2.5 grams
    d. 2.25 grams

14. Rx: Cefazolin 1 gm IVPB q8h. The 2-gm vial states that after reconstitution with 15.5 ml of sterile water, the concentration of the resulting solution is 1 gm/10 ml. What is the powder volume of the vial?

    a. 4.5 ml
    b. 5 ml
    c. 10 ml
    d. 12.5 ml

15. Rx.: Heparin IV @ 1400 units/hr. The IV bag contains NS 1 L with 40,000 units of heparin. Calculate the rate in ml/hr.

    a. 29 ml/hr
    b. 30 ml/hr
    c. 35 ml/hr
    d. 40 ml/hr

16. Dr. Betty Brown writes a prescription for Pam Pennison for Ceclor Susp 20 mg/kg/day po divided q8h × 10 days. Pam is five years old and weighs 48 lb. How much will be given to Pam in each dose if the pharmacy dispenses Ceclor 187-mg/5-ml susp?

    a. 2.5 ml
    b. 3.2 ml
    c. 3.9 ml
    d. 8.6 ml

17. If 80 ml of D70W is infused, how many milligrams of dextrose will the patient receive?

    a. 56 mg
    b. 560 mg
    c. 5600 mg
    d. 56,000 mg

18. Rx: Ceftazidime 3 gm × 9 doses. How many ceftazidime 10-gram vials will the technician need to reconstitute to prepare the 9 doses?

    a. 2
    b. 3
    c. 4
    d. 5

19. A 100-ml IV bag has a strength of 30%. How many grams of solute does this represent?

    a. 3 grams
    b. 1.5 grams
    c. 30 grams
    d. 15 grams

20. How many grams of active ingredient will you need to prepare 2.5 gallons of a 45.6% solution?
    a. 431.49 grams
    b. 4314.9 grams
    c. 43,149 grams
    d. 50,000 grams

21. Doxycycline 100-mg caps cost $23.40/100 caps and the pharmacy applies a 40% markup on cost. What will a patient be charged for 60 caps?
    a. $5.62
    b. $14.04
    c. $19.66
    d. $21.36

22. Rx: Azithromycin 0.5 gm IVPB daily. The 500-mg vial states that the concentration after reconstitution is "250 mg/5 ml." How many milliliters will need to be withdrawn to prepare one dose?
    a. 5 ml
    b. 7.5 ml
    c. 10 ml
    d. 25 ml

23. If you are using 258 ml of hydrochloric acid to prepare a total volume of 2 pints, what is the percentage of hydrochloric acid?
    a. 12.9%
    b. 15.6%
    c. 27.3%
    d. 29.8%

24. What is the percent strength of 1 pint of solution containing 56 g of Camphor?
    a. 84.4%
    b. 53.2%
    c. 13.9%
    d. 11.8%

25. Rx.: Heparin IV @ 2000 units/hr. The IV bag contains NS 1 L with 40,000 units of heparin. The IV set delivers 15 gtt/ml. Calculate the rate in gtt/min.
    a. 9 gtt/min
    b. 10 gtt/min
    c. 13 gtt/min
    d. 15 gtt/min

26. Convert 1:10,000 to a percent strength.
    a. 0.0001%
    b. 0.001%
    c. 0.01%
    d. 0.1%

27. Convert 325 mg to grains.
    a. 4
    b. 5
    c. 6.2
    d. 7

28. Convert 5% to a ratio strength.
    a. 1:2
    b. 1:5
    c. 1:20
    d. 1:50

29. How many milliliters would be given for a 50-mg dose if the available drug has a concentration of 10 mg/5 ml?
    a. 5 ml
    b. 10 ml
    c. 20 ml
    d. 25 ml

30. You need to compound sorbitol 25% 500 ml by mixing sorbitol 70% with sterile water. How much of each will you need?
    a. 321.4 ml of 70% sorbitol and 178.6 ml of sterile water
    b. 250 ml of 70% sorbitol and 250 ml of sterile water
    c. 325 ml of 70% sorbitol and 175 ml of sterile water
    d. 178.6 ml of 70% sorbitol and 321.4 ml of sterile water

14 Math Practice Test II

C omplete this test to review pharmacy calculations.

1. Rx: Diphenhydramine 10-mg/5-ml solution, 500-ml. How much diphenhy-dramine 12.5-mg/5-ml solution will be needed to prepare the prescription?
   a. 100 ml
   b. 200 ml
   c. 350 ml
   d. 400 ml

2. Rx: Allopurinol 300-mg tabs, 450 mg po daily. Dispense: 60 tabs. What is the days' supply for the prescription?
   a. 10
   b. 20
   c. 30
   d. 40

3. Rx: Albuterol oral solution 0.5 mg po tid. Disp: 30-day supply. If the pharmacy dispenses albuterol 2-mg/5-ml solution, how much is needed to fill the prescription?
   a. 1.25 ml
   b. 112.5 ml
   c. 120 ml
   d. 140 ml

4. Rx: Hydrocortisone 0.25% ointment, 120 grams. How many grams of hydrocortisone 2.5% should be mixed with ointment base to prepare the prescription?
   a. 5 grams
   b. 10 grams
   c. 12 grams
   d. 60 grams

5. Furosemide 40-mg tabs cost $23.80/100 tabs and the pharmacy applies a 40% markup on cost plus a $6.50 dispensing fee. What will the patient be charged for 30 tabs?
   a. $16.50
   b. $13.64
   c. $10.00
   d. $7.14

6. How much sorbitol 70% must be mixed with sterile water to prepare 500 ml of sorbitol 10% solution?
   a. 71 ml
   b. 429 ml
   c. 350 ml
   d. 150 ml

7. If the recommended dose of a drug is 500 mg/m^2 per day in two divided doses, how much drug will a patient take in each dose? The patient's BSA = 1.3 m^2.
   a. 125 mg
   b. 250 mg
   c. 325 mg
   d. 650 mg

8. How many teaspoons are in 25 ml?
   a. 1½
   b. 2
   c. 3
   d. 5

9. Order: NS 1 L with 35,000 units of heparin infusing @ 10 ml/hr. Calculate the hourly dosage of heparin.
   a. 350 units/hr
   b. 700 units/hr
   c. 1400 units/hr
   d. 3500 units/hr

10. Rx: Cimetidine 300 mg po qid. Disp: 1-month supply. How many Cimetidine 150-mg tabs are needed to fill the prescription?
    a. 120
    b. 180
    c. 240
    d. 360

11. Rx: Fluoxetine 20 mg po bid. Disp: 90 × 20-mg caps. What is the prescription's days' supply?
    a. 10
    b. 20
    c. 30
    d. 45

12. If the adult dose is 200 mg, what is an appropriate dose for a child weighing 22 kg? (Use Clark's rule.)
    a. 29.3 mg
    b. 64.5 mg
    c. 46.5 mg
    d. 93.2 mg

13. How many grams of NaCl is in two 500-ml bags of D5 NS?
    a. 7.5 grams
    b. 4.5 grams
    c. 2.5 grams
    d. 9 grams

14. Rx: Cefazolin 1.5 gm IVPB q8h. The 2-gm vial states that after reconstitution with 9.5 ml of sterile water, the concentration of the resulting solution is 2 gm/10 ml. What is the powder volume of the vial?
    a. 1.5 ml
    b. 0.5
    c. 10 ml
    d. 2 ml

15. Rx: Heparin IV @ 2100 units/hr. The IV bag contains NS 1 L with 30,000 units of heparin. Calculate the rate in ml/hr.
    a. 35 ml/hr
    b. 50 ml/hr
    c. 60 ml/hr
    d. 70 ml/hr

16. If the adult dose is 250 mg, what is the appropriate dose for a child who weighs 35 lb?
    a. 43.75 mg
    b. 58 mg
    c. 60 mg
    d. 75 mg

17. If 2500 ml of D5W is infused, how many grams of dextrose will the patient receive?
    a. 100 grams
    b. 120 grams
    c. 125 grams
    d. 130 grams

18. Rx: Cefazolin 2 gm IVPB BID. How many cefazolin 10-gram vials will the technician need to reconstitute to prepare a 7-day supply?
    a. 2
    b. 3
    c. 4
    d. 5

19. A 100-ml IV bag has a strength of 70%. How many grams of solute does this represent?
    a. 3 grams
    b. 7 grams
    c. 30 grams
    d. 70 grams

20. How many grams of active ingredient will you need to prepare 500 ml of a 20% solution?
    a. 10 grams
    b. 15 grams
    c. 100 grams
    d. 150 grams

21. Tetracycline 250-mg caps cost $3.40/100 caps and the pharmacy applies a 36% markup on cost + $8.00 dispensing fee. What will a patient be charged for 30 caps?
    a. $1.02
    b. $1.36
    c. $9.02
    d. $9.39

22. Rx: Penicillin 250,000 units IVPB q6h. The 20,000,000-unit vial states that the concentration after reconstitution is "500,000 units/ml." How many milliliters will need to be withdrawn to prepare one dose?
    a. 0.25 ml
    b. 0.5 ml
    c. 1 ml
    d. 1.5 ml

23. If you are using 30 ml of acetic acid to prepare a total volume 120 ml, what is the percentage of acetic acid?
    a. 2.5%
    b. 25%
    c. 40%
    d. 50%

24. What is the percent strength of a 480-ml of solution containing 30 g of active ingredient?
    a. 144%
    b. 62.5%
    c. 14.4%
    d. 6.25%

25. Rx: Heparin IV @ 2500 units/hr. The IV bag contains NS 1 L with 20,000 units of heparin. The IV set delivers 10 gtt/ml. Calculate the rate in gtt/min.
    a. 20 gtt/min
    b. 21 gtt/min
    c. 25 gtt/min
    d. 30 gtt/min

26. Convert 2:20,000 to a percent strength.
    a. 0.0001%
    b. 0.001%
    c. 0.01%
    d. 0.1%

27. Convert 5 mg to mcg.
    a. 0.005 mcg
    b. 5000 mcg
    c. 50 mcg
    d. 0.05 mcg

28. A 20,000,000-unit penicillin vial states that the concentration after reconstitution is "500,000 units/ml." How many milliliters are in the vial after it is reconstituted by the technician?
    a. 10
    b. 20
    c. 40
    d. 50

29. How many milliliters should be given for a 35 mg dose if the available drug has a concentration of 10 mg/ml?
    a. 0.35 ml
    b. 3.5 ml
    c. 7 ml
    d. 8 ml

30. You need to compound 500 ml of sorbitol 10% by mixing 70% sorbitol with sterile water. How much of each will be needed?
    a. 428.6 ml of 70% sorbitol and 71.4 ml of sterile water
    b. 200 ml of 70% sorbitol and 300 ml of sterile water
    c. 325 ml of 70% sorbitol and 175 ml of sterile water
    d. 71.4 ml of 70% sorbitol and 428.6 ml of sterile water

C omplete this test to review pharmacy calculations.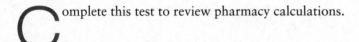

1. Order: Diphenhydramine 75 mg IV q6h. How many diphenhydramine 50-mg/ml, 2 ml mdv, will be needed for a 24-hour supply?

    a. 1
    b. 2
    c. 3
    d. 4

2. Rx: Ampicillin 250 mg caps, 500 mg po q8h × 10 days. How many capsules are needed to fill the prescription?

    a. 30
    b. 60
    c. 50
    d. 40

3. Rx: Docusate sodium oral solution 30 mg po tid. Disp: 30-day supply. If the pharmacy dispenses docusate sodium 50-mg/5-ml solution, how much will the patient take for each dose?

    a. 1.25 ml
    b. 2.5 ml
    c. 3 ml
    d. 3.5 ml

4. Rx: Triamcinolone 0.025% ointment, 120 grams. How many grams of triamcinolone 0.5% will be mixed with an ointment base to prepare the prescription?

    a. 5 grams
    b. 6 grams
    c. 8 grams
    d. 60 grams

5. Amitriptyline 100-mg tabs cost $142.50/1000 tabs and the pharmacy applies a 40% markup on cost plus a $10.50 dispensing fee. What will the patient be charged for 90 tabs?

    a. $190.05
    b. $12.83
    c. $23.33
    d. $28.46

6. How much dextrose 50% must be mixed with sterile water to prepare 2 L of dextrose 10% solution?

   a. 200 mL
   b. 400 mL
   c. 500 mL
   d. 650 mL

7. What is the selling price for a prescription for 30 tablets, if 100 tablets cost $65.30 and the pharmacy applies a 30% markup on cost?

   a. $5.86
   b. $19.59
   c. $24.75
   d. $25.47

8. How many tablespoons are in 450 ml?

   a. 10½
   b. 20
   c. 30
   d. 50

9. Order: NS 500 with 40,000 units of heparin infusing @ 16 ml/hr. Calculate the hourly dosage of heparin.

   a. 350 units/hr
   b. 600 units/hr
   c. 640 units/hr
   d. 1280 units/hr

10. Rx: Ranitidine 150 mg po q12h. Disp: 3-month supply. How many ranitidine 150-mg tabs will be needed to fill the prescription?

    a. 120
    b. 180
    c. 240
    d. 360

11. Rx: Naproxen 500 mg ii po bid. Disp: 60 tabs. What is the prescription's days' supply?

    a. 10
    b. 12
    c. 15
    d. 30

12. If the adult dose is 250 mg, what is an appropriate dose for a six-year-old child? (Use Young's rule.)

    a. 12.5 mg
    b. 38.3 mg
    c. 125 mg
    d. 83.3 mg

13. How many grams of NaCl are in two 1-L bags of D5 ½ NS?

    a. 7.5 grams
    b. 4.5 grams
    c. 2.5 grams
    d. 9 grams

14. Rx: Ceftriaxone 0.5 gm IVPB q12h. The 1-gm vial states that after reconstitution with 8.5 ml of sterile

water, the concentration of the resulting solution is 100 mg/ml. What is the powder volume of the vial?

   a. 1.5 ml
   b. 0.5
   c. 10 ml
   d. 2 ml

15. Rx: Heparin IV @ 1400 units/hr. The IV bag contains NS 1 L with 20,000 units of heparin. Calculate the rate in ml/hr.

    a. 35 ml/hr
    b. 50 ml/hr
    c. 60 ml/hr
    d. 70 ml/hr

16. If the adult dose is 50 mg, what is the appropriate dose for a child who weighs 20 kg?

    a. 14.7 mg
    b. 14.6 mg
    c. 6.7 mg
    d. 6.6 mg

17. If 1000 ml of NS is infused, how many grams of sodium chloride will the patient receive?

    a. 0.45 grams
    b. 0.5 grams
    c. 4.5 grams
    d. 9 grams

18. Rx: Cefazolin 500 mg IVPB q8h. How many cefazolin 10-gram vials will the technician need to reconstitute to batch 100 doses?

    a. 10
    b. 30
    c. 3.3
    d. 5

19. A 100-ml IV bag has a strength of 20%. How many grams of solute does this represent?

    a. 20 grams
    b. 0.2 grams
    c. 30 grams
    d. 70 grams

20. How many grams of active ingredient will you need to prepare 2 L of a 25% solution?

    a. 1500 grams
    b. 1000 grams
    c. 500 grams
    d. 250 grams

21. Ampicillin 250-mg caps cost $69.87/500 caps and the pharmacy applies a 16.2% markup on cost + $15.30 dispensing fee. What will a patient be charged for 40 caps?

    a. $47.77
    b. $21.80
    c. $15.30
    d. $5.59

22. Rx: Penicillin 750,000 units IVPB q6h. The 1,000,000-unit vial states that the concentration after reconstitution is "500,000 units/ml." How many milliliters will need to be withdrawn to prepare one dose?
    a. 0.25 ml
    b. 0.5 ml
    c. 1 ml
    d. 1.5 ml

23. If you are using 90 ml of acetic acid to prepare a total volume of 16 oz, what is the percentage of acetic acid?
    a. 1.87%
    b. 5.3%
    c. 18.8%
    d. 53.3%

24. What is the percent strength of 480-ml of solution containing 69.12 g of active ingredient?
    a. 144%
    b. 62.5%
    c. 14.4%
    d. 6.25%

25. Rx.: D5W @ 120 ml/hr. The IV set delivers 10 gtt/ml. Calculate the rate in gtt/min.
    a. 20 gtt/min
    b. 21 gtt/min
    c. 25 gtt/min
    d. 30 gtt/min

26. Convert 1:15,000 to a percent strength.
    a. 0.006%
    b. 0.007%

c. 0.07%
d. 0.6%

27. Convert 10,000 mcg to mg.
    a. 0.1 mg
    b. 1 mg
    c. 10 mg
    d. 100 mg

28. A 1,000,000-unit penicillin vial states that the concentration after reconstitution is "250,000 units/ml." How many milliliters of penicillin are in the vial after it isreconstituted?
    a. 1
    b. 2
    c. 4
    d. 5

29. How many milliliters should be given for a 35-mg dose if the available drug has a concentration of 5 mg/ml?
    a. 0.35 ml
    b. 3.5 ml
    c. 7 ml
    d. 8 ml

30. You need to compound 2 L of 15% dextrose by mixing 5% dextrose and 20% dextrose. How much of each solution will you need?
    a. 250 ml of 5% dextrose and 750 ml of 20% dextrose
    b. 667 ml of 5% dextrose and 1333 ml of 20% dextrose
    c. 1333 ml of 5% dextrose and 667 ml of 20% dextrose
    d. 750 ml of 5% dextrose and 250 ml of 20% dextrose

chapter 16

Trade/Generic/ Classification Practice Test I

Complete this test to review drug trade name, generic name, and classification knowledge.

1. The generic name for Caduet is
   a. aripiprazole
   b. amlodipine besylate
   c. amlodipine besylate and atorvastatin
   d. amlodipine besylate and benazepril

2. The trade name for dexamethasone is
   a. Desyrel
   b. Dexasone
   c. Diflucan
   d. Deltasone

3. Demadex belongs to which of the following drug classifications?
   a. loop diuretic
   b. analgesic
   c. antihyperlipidemic
   d. skeletal-muscle relaxant

4. The generic name for Abilify is
   a. acyclovir
   b. allopurinol
   c. aripiprazole
   d. azithromycin

5. The generic name for Hyzaar is
   a. losartan
   b. losartan with HCTZ
   c. lovastatin
   d. lisinopril

6. Which of the following is not an ACE inhibitor?
   a. Monopril
   b. Vasotec
   c. Tenoric
   d. Capoten

7. The generic name for Zyrtec is
   a. cephalexin
   b. cetirizine
   c. citalopram
   d. clarithromycin

8. The generic name for Prevacid is
   a. losartan
   b. lansoprazole
   c. lovastatin
   d. lisinopril

9. Which of the following is classified as an antibiotic?
   a. Tussionex
   b. Allegra
   c. Altace
   d. Cipro

10. Which of the following drugs is used to treat salt and water retention associated with congestive heart failure?
    a. ibandronate sodium
    b. ibuprofen
    c. indapamide
    d. indomethacin

11. The trade name for nifedipine is
    a. Pamelor
    b. Paxil
    c. Pepcid
    d. Procardia

12. Which of the following is not an opioid analgesic?
    a. oxycodone
    b. phenobarbital
    c. propoxyphene napsylate
    d. morphine

13. Which of the following drugs is used to treat hypercholesterolemia?
    a. Zocor
    b. Zofran
    c. Zoloft
    d. Zovirax

14. The generic name for Cialis is
    a. travoprost
    b. torsemide
    c. terazosin
    d. tadalafil

15. Which of the following is not used to treat duodenal ulcers?
    a. Pepcid
    b. Zantac
    c. Axid
    d. Vesicare

16. Which of the following is used to treat patients with type II diabetes mellitus?
    a. simvastatin
    b. sitagliptin phosphate
    c. solifenacin succinate
    d. sumatriptan succinate

17. Which of the following drugs is used to treat ADHD?
    a. Flovent
    b. Focalin
    c. Folate
    d. Fosamax

18. Which of the following is not used to treat pyschotic disorders?
    a. ziprasidone
    b. aripiprazole
    c. irbesartan
    d. olanzapine

19. Cyclosporine is the generic name for:
    a. Biaxin
    b. Restasis
    c. Bumex
    d. Namenda

20. Which of the following drugs is used to treat ulcerative colitis?
    a. ibandronate sodium
    b. methotrexate
    c. indapamide
    d. mesalamine

21. Triamcinolone acetonide is a:
    a. CNS stimulant
    b. corticosteroid
    c. muscle relaxant
    d. water-soluble vitamin

22. Norelgestromin and ethinyl estradiol is the generic name for:
    a. Ortho Novum 1/35
    b. Loestrin
    c. Ortho-Cyclen
    d. Ortho Evra

23. Byetta is the trade name for:
    a. eszopiclone
    b. etodolac
    c. exenatide
    d. ezetimibe

24. Which of the following drugs is a calcium channel blocker?
    a. amlodipide
    b. diltiazem
    c. doxazosin
    d. bumetanide

25. Which of the following drugs is not used to treat hyperlipidemia?
    a. ezetimibe
    b. gemfibrozil
    c. felodipine
    d. fenofibrate

26. Fentanyl is the generic name for:
    a. Dolophine
    b. Duoneb
    c. Duragesic
    d. Dyazide

27. Which of the following drugs is not an SSRI antidepressant?
    a. Lexapro
    b. Zoloft
    c. Celexa
    d. Chantix

28. Prempro is the trade name for:
    a. estradiol
    b. conjugated estrogens
    c. medroxyprogesterone
    d. conjugated estrogens and medroxyprogesterone

29. Cephalexin is the generic name for:
    a. Keflex
    b. Keppra
    c. Klonopin
    d. Lamictal

30. Which of the following is used to treat ADHD?
    a. Aricept
    b. Adderall
    c. Ultracet
    d. Atacand

31. Which of the following is used to treat bipolar disorder?
    a. lisinopril
    b. lithium carbonate
    c. lorazepam
    d. losartan

32. Which of the following drugs is used to treat metastatic breast cancer?
    a. Nizoral
    b. Nolvadex
    c. Norvasc
    d. Novolog

33. Which of the following is not an insulin product?
    a. Humalog
    b. Novolin
    c. Lantus
    d. Glycolax

34. Prilosec is the trade name for:
    a. olanzapine
    b. olmesartan
    c. olopatadine
    d. omeprazole

35. Telmisartan is the generic name for:
    a. Mevacor
    b. Micardis
    c. Micronase
    d. Mirapex

36. Which of the following is not a macrolide antibiotic?
    a. Zmax
    b. Biaxin
    c. Minocin
    d. Erythrocin

37. Pamelor is the trade name for:
    a. nortryptyline
    b. minocycline
    c. glyburide
    d. nystatin

38. Atomoxetine is the generic name for:
    a. Singulair
    b. Spiriva
    c. Strattera
    d. Synthroid

39. Which of the following drugs is used in the treatment of bronchospasms associated with COPD?
    a. Diovan
    b. Demadex
    c. Duoneb
    d. Dilantin

40. Clarinex is the trade name for:
    a. desloratadine
    b. loratadine
    c. diphenydramine
    d. dicyclomine

41. Which of the following drugs is used to treat seizures?
    a. Ditropan
    b. Diovan
    c. Dilantin
    d. Diflucan

42. Which of the following is not an oral contraceptive?
    a. Loestrin 24 FE
    b. Kariva
    c. Darvocet-N
    d. Yaz

43. Colace is the trade name for:
    a. divalproex sodium
    b. docusate sodium
    c. docusate calcium
    d. donepezil

44. Verapamil is the generic name for:
    a. Inderal
    b. Indomethacin
    c. Isoptin
    d. Imitrex

45. Which of the following is not a penicillin antibiotic?
    a. Trimox
    b. Augmentin
    c. Veetids
    d. Cipro

46. Which of the following is used to treat diarrhea?
    a. desloratadine
    b. diphenoxylate and atropine
    c. divalproex sodium
    d. docusate sodium

47. Which of the following is the trade name for insuling glargine, rDNA origin?
    a. Lamictal
    b. Lanoxin
    c. Lantus
    d. Lasix

48. Which of the following is not a proton pump inhibitor?
    a. Aciphex
    b. Prilosec
    c. Provigil
    d. Nexium

49. Valium is the trade name for:
    a. diltiazem
    b. digoxin
    c. diclofenac sodium
    d. diazepam

50. Eszopiclone is the generic name for:
    a. Lovaza
    b. Lozol
    c. Lumigan
    d. Lunesta

51. Which of the following drugs is used to treat symptomatic trichomoniasis?
    a. Bentyl
    b. Cogentin
    c. TobraDex
    d. Flagyl

52. Voltaren is the trade name for:
    a. diazepam
    b. diclofenac sodium
    c. dicyclomine
    d. diltiazem

53. Cefdinir is the generic name for:
    a. Keflex
    b. Cefzil
    c. Omnicef
    d. Ceftin

54. Which of the following drugs is used to treat hypertension and symptomatic heart failure?
    a. Vesicare
    b. Voltaren
    c. Viagra
    d. Vasotec

55. Atacand is the trade name for:
    a. carisoprodol
    b. carbidopa
    c. carbamazepine
    d. candesartan cilexetil

56. Doxycycline is the generic name for:
    a. E-mycin
    b. Vibramycin
    c. Zithromax
    d. Sumycin

57. Which of the following is an antifungal drug?
    a. Zyloprim
    b. Allegra
    c. Lotrisone
    d. Reglan

58. Skelaxin is the trade name for:
    a. mesalamine
    b. metaxalone
    c. methadone
    d. methocarbamol

59. Azelastine HCl is the generic name for:
    a. Atarax
    b. Atacand
    c. Astelin
    d. Asacol

60. Which of the following is a CNS stimulant?
    a. metolazone
    b. metoclopramide
    c. methylprednisolone
    d. methylphenidate

61. Benicar is the trade name for:
    a. olmesartan
    b. olanzapine
    c. omeprazole
    d. olopatadine

62. Metoprolol succinate is the generic name for:
    a. Lopressor
    b. Tenormin
    c. Toprol-XL
    d. Lunesta

63. Which of the following drugs is used to treat recurrent ventricular fibrillation?
    a. alendronate sodium
    b. allopurinol
    c. alprazolam
    d. amiodarone

64. Which of the following drugs is used to treat UTI?
    a. phenytoin
    b. niacin
    c. nifedipine
    d. nitrofurantoin

65. Fosinopril sodium is the generic name for:
    a. Minocin
    b. Mirapex
    c. Mobic
    d. Monopril

66. Which of the following is used in the treatment of seizures?
    a. Diflucan
    b. Trileptal
    c. Motrin
    d. Mirapex

67. Adipex-P is the trade name for:
    a. phenytoin sodium
    b. phentermine
    c. phenobarbital
    d. phenazopyridine

68. Oxybutynin chloride is the generic name for:
    a. Ditropan
    b. Dolophine
    c. Drisdol
    d. Duoneb

69. Which of the following is used to treat dry eyes?
    a. fluticasone propionate
    b. hydrocortisone
    c. cyclosporine emulsion
    d. gentamicin

70. Glucophage is the trade name for:
    a. glyburide
    b. metformin
    c. glyburide and metformin
    d. glipizide

71. Which of the following is used to treat bacterial conjunctivitis?
    a. Zocor
    b. Zymar
    c. Zyprexa
    d. Zyrtec

72. Lexapro is the trade name for:
    a. dutasteride
    b. escitalopram
    c. ezetimibe
    d. omeprazole

73. Which of the following is not used to treat erectile dysfunction?
    a. sildenafil citrate
    b. tadalafil
    c. enalapril
    d. verdanafil

74. Combivent is the trade name for:
    a. ipratropium bromide and metoproterenol
    b. ipratropium bromide
    c. salmeterol
    d. ipratropium bromide and albuterol

75. Which of the following is used to treat major depressive disorder?
    a. Effexor
    b. Elavil
    c. Elocon
    d. Estrace

76. Which of the following is not a skeletal-muscle relaxant?
    a. methocarbamol
    b. metaxalone
    c. atomoxetine
    d. carisoprodol

77. Zocor is the trade name for:
    a. sertraline
    b. sildenafil
    c. simvastatin
    d. sitagliptin

78. Tamsulosin is the generic name for:
    a. Flovent
    b. Flomax
    c. Flonase
    d. Tamiflu

79. Which of the following is used to treat spasticity resulting from multiple sclerosis?
    a. Strattera
    b. Lioresal
    c. Zoloft
    d. Imitrex

80. Monteleukast sodium is the generic name for:
    a. Spiriva
    b. Sinequam
    c. Singulair
    d. Seroquel

81. Which of the following drugs is indicated for the treatment of bipolar disorder?
    a. monteleukast sodium
    b. quetiapine fumerate
    c. atomoxetine
    d. rosuvastatin calcium

82. Which of the following drugs is used as a topical analgesic?
    a. Westcort
    b. Nizoral
    c. Lidoderm
    d. Mycolog II

83. Amaryl is the trade name for:
    a. glimepiride
    b. gemfibrozil
    c. glyburide
    d. glipizide

84. Which of the following drugs is used to treat hypothyroidism?
    a. levalbuterol
    b. levetiracetam
    c. levonorgestrel
    d. levothyroxine

85. Which of the following is used to treat glaucoma?
    a. Alphagan
    b. Namenda

c. Cozaar
d. Imdur

86. Lisinopril and HCTZ is the generic name for:
    a. Zestril
    b. Prinzide
    c. Hytrin
    d. Hyzaar

87. Tegretol is the trade name for:
    a. carvedilol
    b. carisoprodol
    c. carbidopa
    d. carbamazepine

88. Which of the following is used to treat rheumatoid arthritis?
    a. Lodine
    b. Zetia
    c. Vytorin
    d. Tricor

89. Plaquenil is used in the treatment/prevention of:
    a. inflammation
    b. hypertension
    c. high cholesterol
    d. malaria

90. Apresoline is the trade name for:
    a. hydroxyzine pamoate
    b. hydralazine
    c. hydroxyzine hcl
    d. hydrocortisone

chapter 17

Trade/Generic/ Classification Practice Test II

Complete this test to review drug trade name, generic name, and classification knowledge.

1. Which of the following drugs is used to treat hypertension and hyperlipidemia?

   a. atenolol and chlorthalidone
   b. amoxicillin and clavulanate potassium
   c. amlodipine besylate and atorvastatin
   d. amlodipine besylate and benazepril

2. The trade name for trazodone is

   a. Desyrel
   b. Dexasone
   c. Diflucan
   d. Deltasone

3. Zetia belongs to which of the following drug classifications?

   a. loop diuretic
   b. analgesic
   c. antihyperlipidemic
   d. skeletal-muscle relaxant

4. Which of the following is used to treat gout?

   a. acyclovir
   b. allopurinol
   c. aripiprazole
   d. azithromycin

5. The generic name for Cozaar is

   a. losartan
   b. losartan with HCTZ
   c. lovastatin
   d. lisinopril

6. Which of the following is an ACE inhibitor?

   a. Avodart
   b. Zestril
   c. Coreg
   d. Aricept

7. The generic name for Celexa is

   a. cephalexin
   b. cetirizine
   c. citalopram
   d. clarithromycin

8. The generic name for Prevacid is
   a. losartan
   b. lansoprazole
   c. lovastatin
   d. lisinopril

9. Which of the following is used to stop coughing?
   a. Tussionex
   b. Allegra
   c. Altace
   d. Cipro

10. The generic name for Motrin is
    a. ibandronate sodium
    b. ibuprofen
    c. indapamide
    d. indomethacin

11. The trade name for bimatoprost is
    a. Lovaza
    b. Lozol
    c. Lumigen
    d. Lyrica

12. Which of the following is used to treat seizures?
    a. oxycodone
    b. phenobarbital
    c. propoxyphene napsylate
    d. morphine

13. The trade name for ondansetron is
    a. Zocor
    b. Zofran
    c. Zoloft
    d. Zovirax

14. The generic name for Demadex is
    a. travoprost
    b. torsemide
    c. terazosin
    d. tadalafil

15. Which of the following is used to treat active duodenal ulcers?
    a. Pepcid
    b. Levsin
    c. Altace
    d. Vesicare

16. Requip is the trade name for:
    a. simvastatin
    b. ropinirole
    c. solifenacin succinate
    d. rosuvastatin

17. Which of the following is used to treat osteoporosis?
    a. Flovent
    b. Focalin
    c. Folate
    d. Fosamax

18. Which of the following drugs is used to treat glaucoma?
    a. glipizide
    b. aripiprazole
    c. irbesartan
    d. latanoprost

19. Which of the following is used in the treatment of short-term anxiety?
    a. Biaxin
    b. Boniva
    c. Bumex
    d. BuSpar

20. Lozol is the trade name for:
    a. ibandronate sodium
    b. ibuprofen
    c. indapamide
    d. indomethacin

21. Methocarbamol is a:
    a. CNS stimulant
    b. corticosteroid
    c. muscle relaxant
    d. water-soluble vitamin

22. Norgestrel and ethinyl estradiol is the generic name for:
    a. Ortho Novum 1/35
    b. Loestrin
    c. Ovral
    d. Ortho Evra

23. Which of the following is used to treat osteoarthritis?
    a. eszopiclone
    b. etodolac
    c. exenatide
    d. ezetimibe

24. Which of the following drug is used to treat edema associated with CHF?
    a. amlodipine
    b. bumetanide
    c. doxazosin
    d. capoten

25. Plendil is the trade name for:
    a. ezetimibe
    b. famotidine
    c. felodipine
    d. fenofibrate

26. Which of the following is used to treat severe pain?
    a. Dolophine
    b. Duoneb
    c. Duragesic
    d. Dyazide

27. Which of the following drugs is used to stop smoking?
    a. Lexapro
    b. Chantix
    c. Celexa
    d. Coumadin

28. Provera is the trade name for:
    a. estradiol
    b. conjugated estrogens
    c. medroxyprogesterone
    d. conjugated estrogens and medroxyprogesterone

29. Which of the following is not used as adjunctive treatment for seizures associated with epilipsy?
    a. Levsinex
    b. Keppra
    c. Klonopin
    d. Lamictal

30. Which of the following is used to treat Alzheimer's disease?
    a. Aricept
    b. Adderall
    c. Ultracet
    d. Atacand

31. Mevacor is the trade name for:
    a. lisinopril
    b. lithium carbonate
    c. lovastatin
    d. losartan

32. Which of the following is used to treat fungal infections?
    a. Nizoral
    b. Nolvadex
    c. Norvasc
    d. Novolog

33. Which of the following is not used to treat diabetes?
    a. Glucovance
    b. Remeron
    c. Januvia
    d. Byetta

34. Which of the following is used in the treatment of allergic conjunctivitis?
    a. olanzapine
    b. olmesartan
    c. olopatadine
    d. omeprazole

35. Pramipexole dihydrochloride is the generic name for:
    a. Mevacor
    b. Micardis
    c. Micronase
    d. Mirapex

36. Which of the following is an anticholinergic?
    a. Levbid
    b. Lantus
    c. Levitra
    d. Lamictal

37. Which of the following is used to treat oral candidiasis?
    a. nortryptyline
    b. minocycline
    c. glyburide
    d. nystatin

38. Which of the following is indicated for prophylaxis and chronic treatment of asthma?
    a. Singulair
    b. Spiriva
    c. Strattera
    d. Synthroid

39. Which of the following is used to treat hypertension?
    a. Diovan
    b. Demadex
    c. Duoneb
    d. Dilantin

40. Which of the following drugs is used to treat irritable bowel syndrome?
    a. desloratadine
    b. loratadine
    c. diphenydramine
    d. dicyclomine

41. Which of the following drugs is used to treat bladder instability associated with voiding in patients with uninhibited neurogenic or reflex neurogenic bladder?
    a. Ditropan
    b. Diovan
    c. Dilantin
    d. Diflucan

42. Which of the following drug is an oral contraceptive?
    a. Benicar
    b. Kariva
    c. Byetta
    d. Imitrex

43. Aricept is the trade name for:
    a. divalproex sodium
    b. docusate sodium
    c. docusate calcium
    d. donepezil

44. Propranolol is the generic name for:
    a. Inderal
    b. Indomethacin
    c. Isoptin
    d. Imitrex

45. Which of the following is a penicillin antibiotic?
    a. Keflex
    b. Augmentin
    c. Minocin
    d. Cipro

46. Which of the following drugs is used to treat manic episodes associated with bipolar disorder?
    a. atropine
    b. diphenoxylate and atropine
    c. divalproex sodium
    d. docusate sodium

47. Which of the following drugs is used to treat mild to moderate heart failure?
    a. Lamictal
    b. Lanoxin
    c. Lantus
    d. Lasix

48. Which of the following is used to treat arrhythmias?
    a. Cordarone
    b. Prilosec
    c. Capoten
    d. Lanoxin

49. Cardizem is the trade name for:
    a. diltiazem
    b. digoxin
    c. diclofenac sodium
    d. diazepam

50. Eszopiclone is the generic name for:
    a. Lovaza
    b. Lozol
    c. Lumigan
    d. Lunesta

51. Which of the following drugs is used to treat parkinsonism?
    a. Bentyl
    b. Cogentin
    c. TobraDex
    d. Flagyl

52. Bentyl is the trade name for:
    a. diazepam
    b. diclofenac sodium
    c. dicyclomine
    d. diltiazem

53. Cefuroxime is the generic name for:
    a. Keflex
    b. Cefzil
    c. Omnicef
    d. Ceftin

54. Which of the following drugs is used to treat erectile dysfunction?
    a. Sertraline
    b. Sildenafil citrate
    c. Simvastatin
    d. Sitagliptin phosphate

55. Which of the following drugs is used to tread musculoskeletal conditions in adults?
    a. carisoprodol
    b. carbidopa
    c. carbamazepine
    d. candesartan cilexetil

56. Tetracycline is the generic name for:
    a. E-mycin
    b. Vibramycin
    c. Zithromax
    d. Sumycin

57. Which of the following drugs is used to treat seasonal allergic rhinitis?
    a. Zyloprim
    b. Allegra
    c. Nizoral
    d. Reglan

58. Asacol is the trade name for:
    a. mesalamine
    b. metaxalone
    c. methadone
    d. methocarbamol

59. Which of the following drugs is used for in the treatment of heart failure in patients with left ventricular systolic dysfunction?
    a. Atarax
    b. Atacand
    c. Astelin
    d. Asacol

60. Which of the following is a corticosteroid?
    a. metolazone
    b. metoclopramide
    c. methylprednisolone
    d. methylphenidate

61. Benicar is the trade name for:
    a. olmesartan
    b. olanzapine
    c. omeprazole
    d. olopatadine

62. Metoprolol tartrate is the generic name for:
    a. Lopressor
    b. Tenormin
    c. Toprol-XL
    d. Lunesta

63. Which of the following drugs is used in the management of anxiety disorders?
    a. amiodarone
    b. allopurinol
    c. alprazolam
    d. alendronate sodium

64. Procardia is the trade name for:
    a. phenytoin
    b. niacin
    c. nifedipine
    d. nitrofurantoin

65. Meloxicam is the generic name for:
    a. Minocin
    b. Mirapex
    c. Mobic
    d. Monopril

66. Which of the following drugs is indicated for vaginal candidiasis?
    a. Diflucan
    b. Trileptal
    c. Motrin
    d. Mirapex

67. Which of the following is used in the treatment of the pain and irritation associated with UTI?
    a. phenytoin sodium
    b. phentermine
    c. phenobarbital
    d. phenazopyridine

68. Vitamin D is the generic name for:
    a. Ditropan
    b. Dolophine
    c. Drisdol
    d. Duoneb

69. Which of the following drugs is used in the prophylactic treatment of asthma?
    a. hydrocortisone
    b. fluticasone propionate
    c. cyclosporine emulsion
    d. gentamicin

70. Glucovance is the trade name for:
    a. glyburide
    b. metformin
    c. glyburide and metformin
    d. glipizide

71. Olanzapine is the generic name for:
    a. Zocor
    b. Zymar
    c. Zyprexa
    d. Zyrtec

72. Which of the following is not used in the treatment of hypertension?
    a. proglitazone
    b. olmesartan medoxomil
    c. fosinopril
    d. candesartan cilexetil

73. Which of the following is used to treat overactive bladder?
    a. tolterodine tartrate
    b. sertraline
    c. enalapril
    d. vardenafil

74. Which of the following drugs is used to reduce very high triglyceride levels in adults?
    a. olmesartan medexomil
    b. ipratropium bromide
    c. omega-E-acid ethyl esters
    d. ipratropium bromide and albuterol

75. Amitriptyline is the generic name for:
    a. Effexor
    b. Elavil
    c. Elocon
    d. Estrace

76. Which of the following is used to treat ADHD?
    a. benazepril
    b. metaxalone
    c. atomoxetine
    d. carisoprodol

77. Januvia is the trade name for:
    a. sertraline
    b. sildenafil
    c. simvastatin
    d. sitagliptin

78. Oseltamivir phosphate is the generic name for:
    a. Osmivir
    b. Flomax
    c. Flonase
    d. Tamiflu

79. Which of the following drugs is used in the treatment of acute migraine attacks?
    a. Strattera
    b. Lioresal
    c. Zoloft
    d. Imitrex

80. Doxepin is the generic name for:
    a. Spiriva
    b. Sinequan
    c. Singulair
    d. Seroquel

81. Crestor is the trade name for:
    a. monteleukast sodium
    b. quetapine fumerate
    c. atomoxetine
    d. rosuvastatin calcium

82. Biaxin is classified as a:
    a. macrolide antibiotic
    b. narcotic analgesic
    c. penicillin antibiotic
    d. tetracycline antibiotic

83. Which of the following is *not* used to improve glycemic control in adults with type II diabetes mellitus?
    a. glimepiride
    b. gemfibrozil
    c. glyburide
    d. glipizide

84. Xopenex is the trade name for:
    a. levothyroxine
    b. levetiracetam
    c. levonorgestrel
    d. levalbuterol

85. Which of the following is used to treat Alzheimer's disease?
    a. Alphagan
    b. Namenda
    c. Cozaar
    d. Imdur

86. Huoscyamine sulfate is the generic name for:
    a. Hytrin
    b. Levsin
    c. Zestril
    d. Hyzaar

87. Which of the following is used to treat mild-to-severe heart failure?
    a. carvedilol
    b. carisoprodol
    c. carbidopa
    d. carbamazepine

88. Which of the following is used to treat high cholesterol levels?
    a. Lodine
    b. Ziac
    c. Vytorin
    d. Ticor

89. Indocin is used in the treatment of:
    a. inflammation
    b. hypertension
    c. high cholesterol
    d. malaria

90. Which of the following drugs is indicated for the treatment of hypertension?
    a. hydroxyzine pamoate
    b. hydralazine
    c. hydroxyzine HCl
    d. hyoscyamine sulfate

Appendix A
Review of Abbreviations and Terminology

A major part of being a successful pharmacy technician is knowing the abbreviations that are commonly used in pharmacy. Although it is not all-inclusive, the following table does list the most common abbreviations you will need to know as a pharmacy technician. Note that as a working pharmacy technician, you may see abbreviations written in a variety of different ways. For example, some abbreviations may be written in all uppercase or in all lowercase letters, with or without periods. In most cases the abbreviations mean the same.

(BID = bid = B.I.D. = b.i.d.)

ABBREVIATION	MEANING
Routes of Administration	
AAA	Apply to affected area
ad	Right ear
AS	Left ear
AU	Both ears
ID	Intradermal
IM	Intramuscular
IPPB	Intermittent positive-pressure breathing (inhalation)
IV	Intravenous or Roman numeral 4
IVP	Intravenous push
IVPB	Intravenous piggyback
NPO	Nothing by mouth
OD	Right eye
OS	Left eye
OU	Each or both eyes
po	By mouth, orally
pr	Rectally
SL	Sublingual
sq, SQ, sc, subq	Subcutaneous
S&S or S/S	Swish and swallow or swish and spit

Schedules	
ā, á	Before
ac	Before meals
ad lib	At liberty, at pleasure
a.m.	Morning
ASAP	As soon as possible
ATC	Around the clock
bid	Twice daily
c̄, ć	With
crm	Cream
d	Day
hr, h	Hour
hs	Bedtime
KVO	Keep vein open
MR	May repeat
MRx1	May repeat 1 time
Noc, N, n	Night
NR, non rep	No refills, no repeat
p	After
pc	After meals
p.m.	Evening
prn	As needed
~~q~~	~~Every~~
qAM	Every morning
qh, q°	Every hour
qhs	Every night at bedtime
qid	Four times daily
~~qod~~	~~Every other day~~
qPM	Every evening
qshift	Every shift
q4h	Every 4 hours
q6h	Every 6 hours
q8h	Every 8 hours
q12h	Every 12 hours
q24h	Every 24 hours

ABBREVIATION	MEANING
s̄	Without
stat	At once, immediately, now
tid	Three times daily
TKO	To keep vein open
ud	As directed
wa	While awake

Dosage Forms

amp	Ampoule
cap(s)	Capsule(s)
CR	Controlled release
DA	Delayed action
DR	Delayed release
DS	Double strength
EC	Enteric-coated
gtt, gtts	Drop, drops
inh	Inhalation or inhaler
inj	Injection
liq	Liquid
MDI	Metered-dose inhaler
ophth	Ophthalmic
otic	Ear
pwd	Powder
SA	Sustained action
soln, sol	Solution
SR	Sustained release
supp	Suppository
susp	Suspension
tab(s)	Tablet(s)
TPN	Total parenteral nutrition
ung, oint	Ointment

IV Solutions

½ NS	Sodium chloride 0.45%
¼ NS	Sodium chloride 0.2% or 0.225%
D5W	Dextrose 5% water
D10W	Dextrose 10% water
D20W	Dextrose 20% water
D30W	Dextrose 30% water
D40W	Dextrose 40% water
D50W	Dextrose 50% water
D70W	Dextrose 70% water
D5 ¼ NS	Dextrose 5% water 0.2% sodium chloride (D5W 0.2% NACL)
D5 ½ NS	Dextrose 5% water 0.45% sodium chloride (D5W 0.45% NACL)
D5NS	Dextrose 5% water 0.9% sodium chloride (D5W 0.9% NACL)
D5LR	Dextrose 5% water and lactated Ringer's (D5WLR)
LR	Lactated Ringer's
NS	Sodium chloride 0.9% (normal saline)

Miscellaneous

@*	At
&	And
ABX	Antibiotic
ad	To, up to
ASO	Automatic stop order
bm	Bowel movement
BP	Blood pressure
CI	Controlled substance— Schedule I
CII	Controlled substance— Schedule II
CIII	Controlled substance— Schedule III
CIV	Controlled substance— Schedule IV
CV	Controlled substance— Schedule V
cc*	Cubic centimeters
Cath	Catheter
Cont	Continue, continuous
CP	Chest pain
CS	Controlled substance
DBP	Diastolic blood pressure
DC, D/C, DC'd	Discontinue, discontinued or discharge, discharged
disp	Dispense

(*Continued*)

ABBREVIATION	MEANING
fs, FS	Floor stock or finger stick
gm	Gram
gr	Grain
HA	Headache
H.O.	House officer
HR	Heart rate
~~I.U.~~	~~International units~~
IVF	Intravenous fluids
L	Liter
LOC	Laxative of choice or loss of consciousness
meds	Medications
mcg	Micrograms
mEq	Milliequivalent
mg	Milligram
ml	Milliliter
mM	Millimole
narc	Narcotic
NGT, Ng tube	Nasogastric tube
NKDA, nka	No known drug allergies, no known allergies
no., #	Number
NTE	Not to exceed
N/V, N&V	Nausea and vomiting
PCA	Patient-controlled analgesic
pt	Patient
qs	Sufficient quantity
qs ad	Sufficient quantity up to
R	Right
Rx	Prescription, take, take thou, recipe
SBP	Systolic blood pressure
Sig	Directions
SOB	Shortness of breath
ss	Half
SZ	Seizure
T, temp	Temperature
T>	Temperature greater than
T<	Temperature less than
tbsp	Tablespoon

tsp	Teaspoon
TO	Telephone order
~~U~~	~~Units~~
USP	United States Pharmacopeia
VO	Verbal order
VS	Vital signs
x	Times or for
µg*	Micrograms
'	Hour
"	Minutes
/	Per, or, and, with
>*	Greater than
<*	Less than
≥	Greater than or equal to
≤	Less than or equal to
↑	Increase
↓	Decrease
Δ	Change
°	hour or degree (24° = 24 hour or 24 degrees)

Chemical Elements

Ag	Silver
Au	Gold
Ca	Calcium
Cl	Chloride
Cu	Copper
Fe	Iron
H	Hydrogen
Hg	Mercury
I	Iodine
K	Potassium
Li	Lithium
Mg	Magnesium
N	Nitrogen
Na	Sodium
O	Oxygen
P	Phosphorus
Zn	Zinc

ABBREVIATION	MEANING
Chemical Compounds	
ACTH	Adrencorticotropic hormone (corticotrophin)
$AgNO_3$	Silver nitrate
APAP	Acetaminophen
ASA	Aspirin
ASA EC	Aspirin, enteric-coated
B_1	Thiamine
B_6	Pyridoxine
B_{12}	Cyanocobalamin
BSS	Balanced salt solution
CaCl	Calcium chloride
$CaCO_3$	Calcium carbonate
D5W	Dextrose 5% in water
DES	Diethylstilbestrol
dig	Digoxin
DPT	Diphtheria, pertussis, tetanus
epi	Epinephrine
ETOH	Ethyl alcohol
$FeSO_4$	Ferrous sulfate
gent	Gentamicin
HBIG	Hepatitis immune globulin
HC	Hydrocortisone
Hcl	Hydrochloride
HCTZ	Hydrochlorothiazide
Hep-lock	Heparin lock flush
H_2O	Water
H_2O_2	Hydrogen peroxide
INH	Isoniazid
IVIG	Intravenous immune globulin
KCL	Potassium chloride
KI	Potassium iodine
KPO_4	Potassium phosphate
L-Dopa	Levodopa
$LiCO_3$	Lithium carbonate
mag cit	Magnesium citrate
MMR	Measles, mump, rubella
MOM	Milk of magnesia
MVI	Multiple vitamins
NaCl	Sodium chloride
$NAHCO_3$, NaBicarb	Sodium bicarbonate
$NaPO_4$	Sodium phosphate
NS	Normal saline
NTG	Nitroglycerin
Pb, Phenobarb	Phenobarbital
PCN	Penicillin
PCN G	Penicillin G
Penicillin VK	Penicillin VK
PO_4	Phosphate
PPD	Purified protein derivative
PTU	Propylthiouracil
SO_4	Sulfate
SSKI	Saturated solution of potassium iodide
tobra	Tobramycin
vit C	Ascorbic acid
vit K	Phytonadione
ZnO	Zinc oxide
$ZnSO_4$	Zinc sulfate

Abbreviations with ~~strikethrough~~ are included in the Joint Commission "DO NOT USE" list and are not supposed to be used in an institutional setting. Also included in the list are the use of a trailing zero (X.0 mg) and lack of a leading zero (.X mg).

Abbreviations followed by an asterisk (*) are being considered for possible inclusion in the "DO NOT USE" list. Also being considered are abbreviations for apothecary units and any abbreviations for drug names.

Pharmaceutical Terminology

Knowledge of terminology is necessary for basic understanding of any language. Review the following terms and definitions as they apply to the pharmacy and medical settings.

A

absorption the time it takes for a drug to work after the drug has been administered; the rate at which the drug passes from the intestines into the bloodstream

active ingredient the chemical in a medication that is known or believed to have a therapeutic effect *acute* refers to a disease or illness with a sudden onset and a short duration

additive a substance added to a liquid solution that is intended for IV use

admixtures a substance that is produced from mixing two or more substances

adverse reaction an unwanted or unexpected side effect or reaction to a medication; may also result from an interaction among two or more medications

aerosol a medication dosage form that contains a gaseous substance consisting of fine liquid or solid particles

alcoholic solution solution that contains only alcohol as the dissolving agent

allergic reaction sensitivity to a specific substance that is contacted through the skin, inhaled into the lungs, swallowed, or injected

allergy a sensitivity of the immune system to a chemical or drug; causes symptoms from rashes to more severe symptoms such as irregular breathing

amphetamines substances that are frequently abused as a stimulant medication; used to treat narcolepsy and eating disorders

analeptic a substance that stimulates the central nervous system

analgesic a substance used to relieve acute or chronic pain

anaphylactic shock a hypersensitivity reaction to another substance

anesthetic a substance that relieves pain by interfering with the nerve transmission that alerts the brain of pain

angiotensin-converting enzyme (ACE) inhibitors used to treat hypertension (high blood pressure) and heart failure by blocking the enzyme that activates angiotensin—a natural substance that narrows the blood vessels, causing high blood pressure

anorectic a substance that suppresses the appetite

antacid a substance that relieves high acid levels in the gastric (stomach) area

antagonist a substance that opposes the action of another drug or substance

antianxiety refers to substances that reduce or relieve anxiety

antibiotic a substance that is used to kill or stop the growth of bacteria in the body

antibody a protein produced by the immune system to respond to foreign substances in the body

anticholinergic a substance that inhibits hypersecretion and gastrointestinal motility

anticoagulant a substance that stops blood clotting (also known as a blood thinner)

anticonvulsant a substance that stops brain nerve firing in order to suppress convulsive seizures

antidepressant a substance that helps maintain proper hormone balance levels to decrease depressive moods

antidiarrheal a substance that relieves and decreases gastrointestinal activity that produces diarrhea

antidote a substance that counteracts the effects of a poisoning agent

antiemetic a substance that relieves nausea and vomiting

antiflatulent a substance that relieves the pressure of excess intestinal gas

antifungal a substance that kills fungus growing in or on the body

antihistamine a substance that stops the effects of histamine release, which cause sneezing, watery eyes, and congestion

antihypertensive a substance that works to lower blood pressure

anti-inflammatory a substance that reduces and relieves inflammation

antineoplastic a substance that is used to kill cancer cells

antioxidant a chemical produced by the body in response to a foreign organism, bacteria, or virus

antiplatelets substances that reduce the ability of platelets to stick together and form a clot

antipruritic a substance that relieves itching

antipsychotics substances that block and inhibit the stimulatory actions of dopamine

antipyretic a substance that relieves and lowers high fever

antispasmodic a substance that relieves stomach-muscle spasms

antitussive a substance that relieves severe cough

antiviral refers to drugs that fight viral infections in the body

aqueous containing water

aseptic techniques techniques that are used to eliminate and protect against bacteria and other microorganisms

astringent a substance that stops secretions or controls bleeding

auxiliary labels labels that are placed on a medication package to provide information and instructions for use

B

beta-blockers substances used in the treatment of hypertension, angina, arrhythmia, and cardiomypathy; may also be used to minimize the possibility of sudden death after a heart attack

binding agent a substance that holds all of the ingredients in a tablet together

bioequivalence refers to a substance that acts on the body with the same strength and similar bioavailability as the same dosage of a sample of a given substance

blood sugar level the measure of glucose (sugar) level in the bloodstream

brand name the proprietary name of a drug, exclusive to a manufacturer for selling and distributive purposes

bronchodilator a substance that relaxes the bronchial smooth muscles in the respiratory system

buccal tablet a tablet that is dissolved in the lining of the cheek rather than swallowed whole

bulk compounding the process of compounding large quantities of a substance for dispensing or distribution

bulk manufacturing the process of manufacturing large quantities of a substance for selling or distribution

bulking agent a chemical substance that is required to produce the desired result

C

calcium channel blockers substances used to treat and reduce hypertension (high blood pressure) and disorders that affect the blood supply to the heart; also used in the treatment of irregular heartbeats

capsule a solid dosage form of a medication that is usually made of gelatin, which holds fine particles of a solid or liquid particle *chewable tablet* tablets that are chewed rather than swallowed whole

chronic refers to a disease or illness that has a long duration (such as for a lifetime)

clinical trial a scientific experiment that tests the effect of a drug in human test patients; required by the FDA for approval of a new medication

communicable refers to a disease or illness that can be transmitted to another person

compound a substance made from a combination of two or more substances

contagious the time period during which an infectious person can transmit the disease to another person through direct or indirect contact

contraindication part of a patient's condition that does not agree with the treatment

controlled-release medications medications that are released and metabolized in the body over a period of time

controlled substance a drug with a high abuse potential; manufacturing and distribution are regulated by the federal government to limit abuse and harm

corticosteroids substances used to prevent minor asthma attacks or to treat severe attacks

cream a dosage form of a medication that is a semisolid preparation, usually applied externally to soothe, lubricate, or protect

cure the effective treatment of a disease or illness, leading to elimination of all symptoms

D

decongestant a substance that shrinks the mucous membranes that cause congestion

dehydration excessive loss of water from the body

diagnosis a process by which a health care professional (doctor, nurse, or technician) determines the patient's condition or disease following tests and examinations

disease a physical process in which the body or specific organs are being destroyed, causing harm and characteristic symptoms to the patient

distribution the process following absorption by which a drug is passed to the cells of various organs

diuretic a substance that increases the water output in the kidneys and reduces water retention in the body

dopamine a neurotransmitter associated with the regulation of movement, emotions, pain, and pleasure

drops a liquid dosage form of medication that is placed in the eye or ear

drug a chemical compound intended for the use in diagnosis, treatment, or prevention of a disease in human or animals; any substance that is intended to produce an alteration to the chemistry and/or functioning in the body

E

effervescent tablet a tablet that is dissolved into a liquid before administration

electrolytes salts that the body requires in its fluids and that are essential in nerve, muscle, and heart functions

elimination the process following distribution by which a drug is broken down and the excess is excreted through the urine

elixir a liquid dosage form that contains flavored water and alcohol mixtures

emulsion a liquid dosage form consisting of a mixture of two products that normally do not mix together

enema a process by which a medicated fluid is injected into the rectum

estrogens hormones that are produced in the ovaries and are responsible for the development and maintenance of female secondary sex characteristics

excretion the process by which the body eliminates waste after metabolism and distribution

expectorant a substance that removes mucus from the upper respiratory system

F

Food and Drug Administration (FDA) the federal agency responsible for the approval, review, and regulation of drugs and dietary supplements

formulary a preferred list of medications that insurance plans allow members to get at a lower out-of-pocket expense

fungicide a substance that kills fungi

G

generic name the nonproprietary name of a drug; also known as the chemical name of the drug

genetically engineered drugs substances that have had foreign genes inserted into their genetic codes artificially

glucagon a hormone produced in the pancreas that causes the automatic release of glucose

glucose the primary energy source and sugar found in the bloodstream

glycogen the principal substance for storing carbohydrates in the body; it is stored in the liver, turned into glucose, and released into the bloodstream when the blood sugar level gets low

H

half-life the amount of time it takes for half of a substance to be broken down in the body and excreted

hazardous waste any substance that is potentially dangerous and toxic to living organisms; must be disposed of properly

health the physical, emotional, or mental well-being of a person

health care procedures, techniques, tests, and examinations that are used to prevent or treat health problems, and maintain a patient's health and well-being

histamine H_2 blockers substances that reduce acid secretion by blocking histamine from reaching the H_2 receptors

hydroalcoholic solution a solution that contains water and alcohol

hypersensitivity an exaggerated response to a given stimulus

hypnotic a substance that relaxes the central nervous system to produce sleep

I

immediate-release medications medications that are released and metabolized immediately following administration

immunosuppressant a substance that is used to prevent the body from rejecting an organ transplant (also known as an antirejection drug)

inactive ingredients the remaining ingredients other than the active ingredient that are found in a drug; used to flavor, digest, color, and bind the whole substance

infusion a slow injection of solution or emulsion into a vein or subcutaneous tissue

inhalation the administration of a medication directly into the lungs by the mouth or nose

inhaler a dosage form that uses a gaseous substance to force fine solid or liquid particles into the respiratory system through the nose or mouth

insulin a hormone secreted by the pancreas that helps the body digest sugars and starches; manufactured insulin is available for use when the pancreas does not produce enough on its own

intolerance an extreme sensitivity to a drug or other substance

intracardiac refers to administration of a medication by injection directly into the heart

intradermal refers to administration of a medication by injection into the skin

intramuscular refers to administration of a medication within or into a muscle

intravenous refers to administration of a medication within or into a vein

inventory the supplies of medications that the pharmacy stocks for dispensing

L

labeling the process of identifying a particular medication with the patient's and physician's information for dispensing

laxative a substance that increases defecation

legend drug a medication that requires a prescription written by a physician before it can be dispensed to a patient

local refers to a small area or single part of the body (for example, a local anesthetic)

lotion a liquid dosage form that contains a powdered substance in a suspension, used externally to soothe, cool, dry, and protect

M

medical devices devices or products used for medical procedures or diagnostic tests

medication order a prescription, usually given in a hospital or other institutional setting

migraine a severe headache caused by extreme changes in the blood vessels in the brain

muscle relaxants substances used to treat involuntary, painful contraction of muscles by slowing the passage to the muscles of nerve signals that cause pain

N

narcotic a drug that is potentially highly abused as a pain reliever, causing dependency and tolerance

narrow therapeutic range the bioequivalence range of a brand drug and its generic counterpart in which very small changes in dosage level could result in toxicity

nonaqueous containing no water

nonlegend drug a medication that does not require a prescription before dispensing; more commonly referred to as an over-the-counter medication

nonsteroidal anti-inflammatory agent a substance that inhibits production of the enzymes that are necessary for the synthesis of prostaglandins, reducing pain and inflammation

O

Occupational Safety and Health Administration (OSHA) the federal agency that is responsible for safety guidelines in the workplace

ointment a semisolid (mixture of a liquid and solid) dosage form that is applied externally to deliver medication, lubricate, and protect

ophthalmic refers to administration of a medication through the eye

opiate a drug that originates from the opium poppy, such as morphine or codeine

opioid a drug, hormone, or other substance that has sedative or narcotic effects similar to substances containing opium or its derivatives

oral refers to administration of a medication by mouth

otic refers to administration of a medication in the ear

overdose an action resulting from ingesting too much of a substance or drug; may result from one dose or multiple doses over the course of time

P

package insert a supplement provided by the manufacturer giving specific details, instructions, and warnings regarding the medication

parenteral refers to administration of medication by any other route than oral; administration by injection

patch a dosage form in which the medication is delivered through a solid application applied to the skin and absorbed into the bloodstream

patent a federally granted, exclusive right to create and sell a product for a specific period of time before other manufacturers can create and sell the identical product

pharmacist a licensed health care professional who is skilled and trained to dispense medications as ordered by a physician and counsel patients on their drug therapies

pharmacokinetics the study of the rates at which drugs are metabolized, distributed, and excreted from the body after consumption

pharmacology the study of drugs and their effects on the body

placebo a pill-like preparation that contains no active or chemical ingredient, usually given for its psychological effects (commonly referred to as a sugar pill)

prescription a direction given by a physician for the preparation and use of a medication for a specific patient to be dispensed by a pharmacist

progestin a female reproductive hormone that causes menstruation as it triggers the shedding of the uterine lining

proton pump inhibitor a substance that reduces gastric acid buildup by blocking the release of protons by proton pumps

psychotherapeutic drugs substances that are used to relieve the symptoms of mental and psychiatric illnesses, such as depression, psychosis, and anxiety

psychotropic a substance that affects a person's ability to distinguish reality from imagination

R

recreational drugs drugs (usually illegal) that are often used in a social setting for their pleasurable effects rather than medicinal value

rectally refers to administration of a solid or liquid medication through the rectum

S

Schedule I drugs drugs classified by the Drug Enforcement Agency as having ahigh abuse potential and with no FDA approval for medicinal use (illegal drugs)

Schedule II drugs drugs classified by the Drug Enforcement Agency as having high abuse potential with severe dependence liability (narcotics, amphetamines, stimulants)

Schedule III drugs drugs classified by the Drug Enforcement Agency as having less abuse potential than Schedule II drugs and moderate dependence liability (non-narcotic stimulants, nonbarbituate sedatives, anabolic steroids)

Schedule IV drugs drugs classified by the Drug Enforcement Agency as having less abuse potential than Schedule III drugs and limited dependence liability (sedatives, antianxiety agents, non-narcotic analgesics)

Schedule V drugs drugs that have limited abuse potential; available as prescription or over-the-counter drugs (cough syrups with small amounts of codeine, antitussives, antidiarrheals)

sedative a substance that relieves anxiety and tension; calms and relaxes

side effect a predicted, unwanted reaction to a substance or combination of substances

slow-release medication a medication that is released and metabolized in the body over a period of time

solution a liquid dosage form in which the medication is completely dissolved in a liquid

sterilize to cleanse objects, wounds, burns, and so on, of microorganisms such as bacteria

stimulants a class of medications that are intended to increase alertness and physical activity

subcutaneous refers to administration of a medication under the skin

sublingual tablet a tablet that is dissolved under the tongue rather than swallowed whole

suppository a solid medication given through the vagina or rectum

suspension a liquid dosage form in which the solid particles are not completely dissolved

symptom a condition that usually comes before the onset of a disease or illness; an abnormality that indicates the existence of a disease or illness

syrup a liquid dosage form that consists of water and sugar mixed with the medication

T

tablet a solid dosage form in which the ingredients are compacted into a small, formed shape

tolerance the condition in which the body has become unresponsive to a substance after prolonged exposure

topical refers to a substance used externally for relief of swelling, itching, or infection

transdermal refers to administration of a medication through the skin (for example, patches)

U

U.S. Pharmacopeia (USP) a nonprofit organization, recognized by the FDA, that publishes standards on prescription drugs, over-the-counter medications, dietary supplements, and health care products

V

vaginal tablet a tablet that is dissolved in the mucous lining of the vagina

vaginally refers to administration of a solid or liquid medication through the vagina

vasodilator a substance that causes the blood vessels to widen

W

withdrawal symptom an effect that occurs with sudden stopping of the use of a substance after prolonged use

Medical Terminology

A

acne vulgaris a skin condition that occurs as a result of the overproduction of oil by the oil glands of the skin and results in pimples, blackheads, and whiteheads on the surface of the skin

addiction physical or psychological dependence on a chemical substance such as alcohol; refers to any habit that cannot easily be given up

amnesia loss of memory (may be short- or long-term)

anatomy the study of the structures in living things

anemia a condition in which there are very few red blood cells in the bloodstream that can carry oxygen to the tissues

anesthesiologist a physician who specializes in administering drugs to anesthetize or sedate patients before a surgical procedure and who monitors a patient's vital signs while under anesthesia

angina pectoris a condition characterized by an attack of chest pain caused by an insufficient supply of oxygen to the heart

anorexia an eating disorder characterized by a refusal to maintain body weight in a healthy range, low self-esteem, and an intense fear of gaining weight

arrhythmia an irregular heartbeat

arteriosclerosis a condition characterized by thickening and hardening of the arteries

arthritis a condition characterized by inflammation of the joints

asthma a condition that affects the breathing of a patient by restricting the airway and oxygen supply as a result of inflammation, swelling, and irritation

attention-deficit disorder (ADD) a mental disorder characterized by developmentally inappropriate levels of attention, concentration, activity, distractibility, and impulsivity

attention-deficit hyperactivity disorder (ADHD) a mental disorder characterized by impulsive behavior, difficulty concentrating, and hyperactivity that affects social, academic, or occupational functioning

autoimmune disorder a disorder characterized by an immune response against the body's own tissues

B

bacteria single-celled microorganisms that are abundant in most living things; may be beneficial or cause harm to a person

benign refers to a condition or abnormal growth that is not cancerous (such as a tumor or cyst)

blood pressure the force exerted by blood against the walls of the arteries; measured when the heart contracts and relaxes

bloodstream the area in which the blood flows through the capillaries, veins, and arteries

body mass index (BMI) a measurement of body fat based on the patient's height and weight

bronchitis acute inflammation of the bronchial tubes in the lungs

C

carcinogen any agent capable of causing cancer

cardiologist a physician who specializes in the treatment of cardiac (heart) disorders and illnesses

cardiovascular disease conditions of the heart and circulation system

catalyst a substance that speeds up a chemical reaction without being changed or destroyed by the reaction

cavity a hollow space in a structure

cerebral refers to the brain

chemotherapy prevention or treatment of cancerous disease by using toxic chemical agents

cholesterol a substance produced in the liver and necessary for normal functioning of the body, including production of hormones, bile, and vitamin D

clinical refers to diagnostic tests, labs, and procedures that require close observation of patients

congestive heart failure a potentially fatal condition of the cardiovascular system in which the heart has lost its ability to pump blood in and out

contraceptives drugs and devices used for the prevention of pregnancy; can also be used for hormone regulation

cranial refers to the skull or head

cystitis inflammation of the urinary bladder

D

dementia a disease characterized by progressive memory loss and by learning and thinking disorders; often leads to Alzheimer's disease

dependency physical and/or psychological reliance on a chemical substance or habit

depression a mental disorder in which the person feels sad and helpless; characterized by personality changes and a loss of socialization, communication, and energy

dermatologist a physician who specializes in the treatment of skin disorders and illnesses

detoxification a process in which a patient is medically supervised during withdrawal from alcohol or drug dependency

diabetes a condition characterized by lack of insulin production in the pancreas, which is essential for digesting and retrieving energy from food

distal refers to a body part that is farthest from the point of attachment

E

edema abnormal swelling caused by a buildup of fluids in tissues and organs

emergency medicine specialist a physician who specializes in the treatment of emergency situations and trauma

emphysema an irreversible disease caused usually by long-term smoking, in which there has been severe damage to the alveoli (tiny air sacs) in the lungs, resulting in a decrease in the exchange of gases; results in wheezing, coughing, and shortness/difficulty of breath

endorphin a chemical or ingredient produced by the body that relieves pain and stress

erythrocyte a red blood cell

esophagitis inflammation of the esophagus as a result of acid buildup

euphoria a feeling of great happiness and well-being

excretion the process by which waste is eliminated from the body

external refers to the outer or outside part of a structure

G

gastric ulcer a tear in the normal tissue lining of the stomach wall

gastritis inflammation of the normal tissue lining of the stomach wall

gastroenterologist a physician who specializes in the treatment of digestive disorders and illnesses

gastroesophageal reflux disease (GERD) a condition that occurs when incompletely digested food is forced back up the esophagus; the food is very acidic and irritates the esophagus, causing heartburn and other symptoms

gastrointestinal tract the part of the digestive system that includes the mouth, esophagus, stomach, and intestines; aids in digesting and processing food in the body

geriatric refers to the care and treatment of elderly patients

glaucoma an eye condition caused by a buildup of pressure caused by reduced drainage of fluid from the eye, possibly resulting in loss of vision

gynecologist a physician who specializes in the treatment of disorders of the female reproductive organs

H

heartburn a painful burning sensation in the esophagus, just below the breastbone

hemorrhage severe, uncontrollable bleeding (may be external or internal)

hepatitis inflammation of the liver

herpes simplex an acute viral disease characterized by watery blisters on the skin and mucous membranes; commonly known as cold sores

hormone a chemical substance that stimulates and regulates certain bodily functions

hormone replacement therapy (HRT) a therapy developed for women to help increase the declining amounts of estrogen caused by menopause

hyperglycemia high blood glucose (sugar)

hyperlipidemia high cholesterol

hypertension long-term high blood pressure

hypoglycemia low blood glucose (sugar)

I

immunity the body's ability to fight off infections from bacteria and viruses

impotence the inability to achieve and maintain penile erection

inflammation redness, swelling, pain, and heat in a body tissue(s) caused by physical injury, infection, or irritation

influenza a contagious viral infection of the nose, throat, and lungs that often occurs in the winter season

inpatient a person who has been admitted to a hospital or other medical facility to receive treatment for a disease

internal refers to the inner or inside part of a structure

L

leukemia a condition characterized by high white blood cell counts

leukocyte a white blood cell

lipids organic compounds consisting of fats and other substances; used to measure cholesterol

M

malignant refers to an abnormal condition or growth in which a group of cells causes harm and destruction to other cells and tissues (for example, cancerous cells)

metabolism the physical and chemical processes of the body that convert consumed food into energy for use by the tissues and organs

metastasis the spreading of a disease from one organ to another organ or part of the body

N

narcolepsy a rare, chronic sleep disorder characterized by constant daytime fatigue and sudden attacks of sleep

nausea a feeling of sickness in the stomach, usually accompanied by the urge to vomit

neurologist a physician who specializes in the treatment of disorders and illnesses of the brain and central nervous system

neuropathic refers to a disease of the nerves

neurotransmitter a substance released by one nerve cell that activates or inhibits a neighboring nerve cell

O

obstetrician a physician who specializes in the care of pregnant women before and during the birth of babies

oncologist a physician who specializes in the treatment of cancer

ophthalmologist a physician who specializes in the treatment of poor vision and eye disorders with medication, corrective lenses, and surgery

organ a part of the body made up of tissues that performs a specialized function; part of an organ system

orthopedist a physician who specializes in the treatment of injuries and structural disorders of the bones and joints

osteoporosis a loss in total bone density that may result from calcium deficiency, menopause, certain endocrine diseases, advanced age, medications, or other risk factors

otolaryngologist a physician who specializes in the treatment of disorders and illnesses of the ear, nose, and throat

outpatient refers to patients who receive treatment from a hospital or other medical facility on a scheduled basis without being admitted for overnight or continuous stay

P

pain a feeling of slight or severe discomfort caused by an injury or illness

panic attack a sudden, repeated episode of extreme fear, panic, and anxiety

parietal refers to the wall of a structure

pathogen a microorganism that causes a disease (bacteria or virus)

pathologist a physician who studies the history, causes, and progress of diseases by examining specimens of body tissues, blood, fluids, and secretions

pathology the study of the nature of disease

peripheral at or toward the surface of the body or its parts

physiology the study of the function of living things

prevention taking steps before a health condition or other abnormality occurs or worsens

primary care the medical care a person receives from a general practitioner or family physician

primary care physician usually an internal medicine or family physician who can treat a variety of illnesses; refers a patient to a specialist if further specialized care or treatment is necessary

prognosis medical assessment of the expected outcome and course of a particular disease

proximal refers to a body part that is nearest to the point of attachment

psychiatrist a physician who specializes in the treatment of mental, emotional, and behavioral disorders; uses medications and psychotherapy

psychotherapy nondrug treatment of psychological disorders performed as behavioral or cognitive therapy

pulmonary refers to the lungs and respiratory system

R

radiologist a physician who uses technologies such as X-rays, radiation therapy, and ultrasound machines to view, analyse, and treat medical problems

receptor part of the nerve cell that recognizes a neurotransmitter and communicates with other nerve cells

respiration the process by which gases are passed through the lungs and distributed throughout the body

S

seasonal affective disorder (SAD) a type of depression that occurs during the fall and winter months only

secondary care the medical care a person receives from a specialist after being referred by his or her primary physician

serotonin a neurotransmitter in the brain that functions to regulate moods, appetite, sensory perception, and other central nervous system functions

spasm an involuntary muscle contraction

specialist a physician who is experienced in a certain area of study for treatment and prevention *surgeon* a physician who is trained to perform surgical procedures and operations on patients in order to provide treatment or cure for an illness

syndrome a set of symptoms that are characteristic of a particular disease

systemic refers to the whole body

T

terminally ill the condition of having an illness or disease for which there is no treatment or cure available; expected result of the disease is death

testosterone a hormone produced in high amounts in males that regulates certain characteristics of muscle building, sexual organs, hair growth, and the deepening of the voice during puberty

toxic refers to a poisonous substance

U

urinary incontinence the inability to control the holding of urine in the bladder

urologist a physician who specializes in the treatment of disorders of the urinary tract, as well as problems in the male reproductive organs

V

vaccine a preparation that contains killed or weakened viruses or bacteria, which is administered to a person to provide active immunity against a disease

vascular refers to the blood vessels and circulatory system

vertigo a condition characterized by dizziness

virus very small infectious organisms that require a living cell to reproduce

visceral refers to the structures inside the body

Appendix B
Professional Resources

Reference Books

Clinical Books

- *American Hospital Formulary Service Drug Information (AHFS)*
- *Drug Facts and Comparisons*
- *Drug Handbook for the Allied Health Professional*
- *Martindale's*
- *Physician's Drug Reference* (paid for by drug manufacturers)

Product Information

American Drug Index
First Data Bank

Pharmaceutical Management

Applied Therapeutics: The Clinical Use of Drugs
Manual of Therapeutics
Merck Manual

Certification/Accreditation/ Regulations

ACPE—Accreditation Council for Pharmacy Education

www.acpe-accredit.org
312-664-3575 (phone)
312-664-4652 (fax)
20 North Clark Street, Suite 2500
Chicago, IL 60602-5109

ExCPT—Exam for the Certification of Pharmacy Technicians

www.nationaltechexam.org
314-442-6775
2536 S. Old Hwy 94
Suite 224
St. Charles, MO 63303

NABP—National Association of Boards of Pharmacy

www.nabp.net
847-391-4406 (phone)
847-391-4502 (fax)
1600 Feehanville Drive
Mount Prospect, IL 60056

PTCB—Pharmacy Technician Certification Board

www.ptcb.org
800-363-8012 (phone)
202-429-7596 (fax)
2215 Constitution Avenue, NW
Washington, DC 20037-2985

National Associations

AAPT—American Association of Pharmacy Technicians

www.pharmacytechnician.com

APhA—American Pharmacists Association

www.aphanet.org
202-628-4410 / 800-237-2742 (phone)
202-783-2351 (fax)
2215 Constitution Avenue, NW
Washington, DC 22037

ASHP—American Society of Health-System Pharmacists

www.ashp.org
301-657-3000 / 866-279-0681 (phone)
7272 Wisconsin Avenue
Bethesda, MD 20814

CAPT—Canadian Association of Pharmacy Technicians

www.capt.ca
416-410-1142 (phone)
15-6500 Millcreek Drive, Suite #165
Mississauga, ON L5N 3E7

NACDS—National Association of Chain Drug Stores

www.nacds.org
703-549-3001 (phone)
413 North Lee Street
Alexandria, VA 22314

NACP—National Community Pharmacists Association

www.ncpanet.org
703-683-8200 / 800-544-7447 (phone)
703-683-3619 (fax)
100 Daingerfield Road
Alexandria, VA 22314

NPTA—National Pharmacy Technician Association

www.pharmacytechnician.org
888-247-8700 (phone)
888-247-8706 (fax)
PO Box 683148
Houston, TX 77268

PTEC—Pharmacy Technician Educators Council

www.rxptec.org

Other

APHA—American Public Health Association

www.apha.org

CDC—Centers for Disease Control

www.cdc.gov

DEA—U.S. Drug Enforcement Administration

www.dea.gov

FDA—U.S. Food & Drug Administration

www.fda.gov

RxList

www.rxlist.com

USP—United States Pharmacopeia

www.usp.gov

WebMD

www.webmd.com

Appendix C
Answers

Ch. 1 Review Questions

1. d	2. a	3. e	4. d	5. b
6. d	7. b	8. d	9. a	10. a

Ch. 2 Review Questions

1. b	2. b	3. c	4. e	5. b
6. d	7. b	8. c	9. b	10. d
11. e	12. c	13. c	14. a	15. c
16. c	17. d	18. a	19. b	20. c

Ch. 3 Review Questions

1. d	2. d	3. b	4. c	5. b
6. a	7. c	8. c	9. b	10. c

Ch. 4 Review Questions

1. b	2. d	3. b	4. b	5. d
6. c	7. a	8. b	9. c	10. d

Ch. 5 Review Questions

1. a	2. b	3. d	4. d	5. c
6. b	7. e	8. a	9. d	10. c

Ch. 6 Review Questions

1. c	2. a	3. b	4. d	5. d
6. c	7. b	8. d	9. b	10. b

Practice Certification Exam I

1. d. $\dfrac{1400\ mL}{12\ hr} \times \dfrac{40\ gtt}{1\ mL} \times \dfrac{1\ hr}{60\ min} = \dfrac{56{,}000\ gtt}{720\ min}$
$= 77.7\ gtt/min$

Round up to 78 gtt/min.

2. b. Enalapril is an ACE inhibitor.

3. c. $\dfrac{76.78}{100} = \dfrac{X}{30}$

$100x = 76.78 \times 30$

$100x = 2303.4$

$x = 23.03$ (AWP for 30 tabs)

$\underline{+\ 7.75}$ (Dispensing Fee)

$\$30.78$ Total for 30 tabs

4. c. Because methylphenidate is a Schedule II drug, it cannot be written with refills.

5. b. A technician should always forward questions of this nature to the pharmacist, because technicians cannot legally counsel patients.

6. a. Diphenhydramine is the generic name for Benadryl.

7. b.

2.5		0.5
	1.5	
1		1

Total

Parts 1.5

$\dfrac{0.5}{1.5} \times 60 = 20$ g of 2.5%

$\dfrac{1}{1.5} \times 60 = 40$ g of 1%

The correct answer is 40 g of 1% and 20 g of 2.5%.

8. d. Whenever an investigational drug is used, a physician must initiate the order for the drug.

9. b. $\dfrac{3}{100} = \dfrac{x}{150}$

$100x = 450$

$x = 4.5$ gm

4.5 gm $\times 1000$ mg/gm $= 4500$ mg

$\dfrac{500\ mg}{tab} = \dfrac{4500\ mg}{x}$

$500x = 4500$ mg

$x = 9$ tablets

10. d. An antipyretic is indicated to reduce fever.

11. b. medication name and strength, lot number, and expiration date

12. c. $\dfrac{250\ mg}{5\ mL} = \dfrac{400\ mg}{x\ mL}$

$250 \times x = 5 \times 400$

$250x = 2000$

$x = 8$ mL

Each dose will be 8 mL. 8 mL tid for 10 days equals 240 mL total volume needed.

13. b. A Luer-Loc syringe should always be used when mixing hazardous medications.

14. b. Lortab is classified as a Schedule III controlled substance.

15. d. Inventory turnover refers to how often medications are used and reordered.

16. b. The co-payment is the portion of the retail price that the patient must pay.

17. d. 42 capsules will be needed to give a patient 1 capsule tid for 14 days.

18. b. Prescription medications are also called legend drugs.

19. c. Stock rotation consists of always keeping the shortest expiration dates to the front of the shelf, to ensure that they are dispensed first.

20. a. The drug propranolol is classed as a beta-blocker.

21. b. $\dfrac{2 \text{ mEq}}{\text{ml}} = \dfrac{8 \text{ mEq}}{x \text{ ml}}$

$2x = 8$

$x = 4$ ml

22. b. An invoice is the wholesaler's bill to the pharmacy, and it is used by the pharmacy when paying for the drug order.

23. c.

10		3
	5	
2		5

Total

Parts 8

$\dfrac{3}{8} \times 120 = 45$ grams of 10%

$\dfrac{5}{8} \times 120 = 75$ grams of 2%

24. a. 2–8°C equals 36–46°F, which is the required temperature for storage under refrigeration.

25. d. A phone call is not considered a direct copy. A nurse or a pharmacist may receive a telephoned order from a physician, but a nurse cannot simply call an initial order to the pharmacy. The written documentation of the order must be reviewed by a pharmacist before it can be filled.

26. b. $\dfrac{5}{100} = \dfrac{x}{300}$

$x = 15$

27. b. Confidentiality protects identity and health information of patients from those who are not authorized to have such information.

28. c. Any controlled substance in Schedule III, IV, or V may be refilled up to five times within 6 months after the prescription is written.

29. b. The four-digit group in an NDC number signifies the drug product.

30. d. Glucotrol is the trade name for glipizide.

31. a. 125 ml/hr × 24 hr = 3000 ml

32. c. 164 lb/2.2 = 74.5 kg

74.5 kg × 5 mg = 372.5/day

372.5 mg/3 doses = 124.2 mg/dose

This will round down to 124 mg/dose.

33. b. Ranitidine is classed as an H_2 antagonist.

34. d. Because furosemide is a non–potassium-sparing diuretic, it causes loss of potassium along with the fluid that is lost. Potassium supplements are usually given in conjunction with a drug of this nature.

35. d. Lisinopril and glyburide are the generic names for Prinivil and Diabeta.

36. c. $\dfrac{0.5}{100} = \dfrac{x}{60}$

$100x = 30$

$x = 0.3$ gram

0.3 gram × 1000 mg/gram = 300 mg

37. b. 2 tabs po q4–6h prn coincides with the directions given.

38. a.

15%		5
	10%	
5%		5

The ratio 5:5 can be reduced to a 1:1 ratio.

39. c. Doxycycline, a tetracycline derivative, can make the skin especially sensitive to the sun. This condition is known as photosensitivity.

40. d. First convert 2 g to milligrams by multiplying by 1000 (1 g = 1000 mg). Then 2000 mg divided by 250 mg (each dose) = 8 doses.

41. d. Nitroglycerin should always be stored in its original container, which is air-tight and light-resistant. Exposure to light will decrease the potency of the nitroglycerin over a period of time.

42. c. The blower on the laminar airflow workbench should run for at least 30 minutes before use to ensure that the air within the hood meets the standards of ISO5.

43. b. The 18-gauge needle has the largest bore. (Hint: The smaller the number, the bigger the needle.)

44. a. A "No alcohol" auxiliary label should always be placed on the container when dispensing metronidazole to a patient. Consuming alcohol while using this drug will cause an antabuse-type reaction, including severe nausea and profuse vomiting.

45. b. 500 mL × 15% = 1500 mL × x%

500 × 0.15 = 1500 × x

75 = 1500x

0.05 = x

5% = x

46. b. Instill 3 drops in the left ear three times daily as needed for pain.

47. c. A patient who is allergic to penicillin has a 1-in-10 chance of being allergic to a cephalosporin. This is known as cross-sensitivity.

48. b. $\dfrac{1}{2}$ gr = 30 mg

49. b. $$\frac{1000 \text{ mL}}{12 \text{ hr}} \mid \frac{15 \text{ gtt}}{1 \text{ mL}} \mid \frac{1 \text{ hr}}{60 \text{ min}}$$

    $$= \frac{15,000 \text{ gtt}}{720 \text{ min}} = 20.83 \text{ gtt/min}$$

    Round up to 21 gtt/min.

50. a. Inspections every six months are required to ensure that the laminar airflow workbench is working properly.

51. c. Zovirax and Epivir are both antiviral agents. (Hint: *vir* is in both drug names.)

52. b. $$\frac{40 \text{ mEq}}{1000 \text{ mL}} = \frac{x \text{ mEq}}{80 \text{ mL}}$$

    (Hint: 1 L = 1000 mL.)

    $$40 \times 80 = 1000 \times x$$
    $$3200 = 1000x$$
    $$3.2 \text{ mEq} = x$$

    There are 3.2 mEq in 80 mL, and the patient will receive 80 mL/hr. Therefore, the patient will receive 3.2 mEq of KCl per hour.

53. d. Na is the chemical symbol for sodium.

54. d. A 5-micron filter needle will be sufficient to filter out tiny glass fragments from an opened ampoule.

55. b. Rifampin is used to treat tuberculosis.

56. d. The volume of liquid is always read at the bottom of the meniscus.

57. c. $$\frac{2}{100} = \frac{1}{x}$$
    $$2x = 100$$
    $$x = 50$$

58. b. The Poison Prevention Packaging Act of 1970 states that child-resistant caps should be used on all dispensing containers unless the drug is exempt or the patient requests otherwise.

59. c. 180 mL = 6 oz. (Hint: 30 mL = 1 oz.)

60. b. 142 lb ÷ 2.2 (2.2 lb = 1 kg) = 64.5 kg

    15 mg × 64.5 kg = 968.1 mg/day

    968.1 divided by ÷ 3 (number of equal doses)

    = 322.7 mg/dose

    Round up to 323 mg.

61. b. The FDA's MedWatch form is used to report any adverse drug reactions.

62. c. Pepcid and Zantac are both H_2 antagonists.

63. c. $4.50 × 30% = $1.35

    $4.50 + $1.35 = $5.85

64. b. Tetracycline and tetracycline-derivative drugs should never be administered with antacids or dairy products. This medication will bind to the antacids or dairy products and simply pass through without being absorbed systemically.

65. c. Temazepam is classed as a Schedule IV drug, as are most sedatives and hypnotics.

66. d. 15–30°C is equivalent to 59–86°F. This is the correct temperature for room-temperature storage.

67. b. A formulary is a list of accepted medications from which a physician may prescribe. This formulary is standardized and approved by the pharmacy and therapeutics (P&T) committee.

68. d. Any information that could identify a patient is considered protected health information under HIPAA.

69. d. Vinblastine is a chemotherapeutic agent and therefore should be handled as a hazardous medication. A spill kit should be used to clean the area if a spill/breakage occurs.

70. c. When cleaning the laminar airflow workbench, always clean the hanging bar and sides first. When cleaning the sides, clean from top to bottom, working outward from the filter. Always clean the work surface last. Never spray anything directly onto the HEPA filter, because doing so could weaken or damage it.

71. b. 120 mL × 0.05% = x mL × 5%
    $$120 \times 0.0005 = x \times 0.05$$
    $$0.05 = 0.05x$$
    $$1.2 = x$$

72. b. Ampicillin injection should always be diluted with normal saline for best stability. If mixed with dextrose, stability is greatly diminished.

73. b. 60 ml/hr × 20 hours = 1200 ml total volume needed. 1 L = 1000 mL; therefore, two bags will be sufficient to complete the 20-hr infusion.

74. a. The packing slip is used by the wholesaler to pull the drug order in the warehouse. The packing slip accompanies the drug order to the pharmacy.

75. d. $$200 \text{ mL} \times \frac{1}{200} = 500 \text{ mL} \times x\%$$
    $$200 \times 0.0005 = 500 \times x$$
    $$0.1 = 500x$$
    $$0.0002 = x$$
    $$0.02\% = x$$

76. c. A secondary infusion attached to a main IV line is called a piggyback.

77. c. Federal law requires records to be kept for a minimum of 2 years.

78. a. The 000 is the largest size empty gelatin capsule used in extemporaneous compounding. (Hint: The smaller the number, the larger the capsule.)

79. b. When working in the laminar airflow workbench, all manipulations should be at least 6 inches within the hood.

80. a. Amlodipine is classed as a calcium channel blocker.

81. c. A want book is a list of items that need to be ordered when using a manual inventory system.

82. c. The second letter corresponds to the first letter of the prescriber's last name.

    Add $1 + 5 + 6 = 12$

    Add $3 + 5 + 7 = 15 \times 2 = 30$

    Add $12 + 30 = 42$

    2 is the check digit, so this is the only number that could be a valid DEA number.

83. c. A Class III drug recall is the least severe of all recall classes. This type of recall is not likely to cause harm to the patient.

84. b. A DEA Form 222c is used to order Schedule II controlled substances.

85. d. Controlled substances, investigational drugs, and chemotherapy drugs all require special handling. Check your pharmacy P&P for specifics.

86. a. The Orange Book is most often used to find generic equivalent drugs.

87. d. Nursing station inspections are a responsibility of the pharmacy technician and are performed to ensure that drugs are being stored and used correctly in patient care areas.

88. b. Warfarin and aspirin used together without a doctor's approval and appropriate monitoring could result in hemorrhage, since both of these drugs are anticoagulants. This could be a major drug–drug interaction.

89. b. 35 units + 15 units = 50 units/day

    50 units $\times$ 30 days = 1500 units/30 days

    Since each vial of insulin holds 1000 units, the patient will need two vials.

90. d. Nitroglycerin tablets and injections should always be dispensed in the original glass container. If it is dispensed in a plastic container, the medication may adhere to the plastic.

Practice Certification Exam II

1. b. The Automix is used for TPN compounding, the PhaSeal for chemotherapy preparation, and the Pyxis and MedCarousel for medication dispensing.

2. b. A tablet can be prepared by either compression or molding.

3. d. The trade for ramipril is altace.

4. c. Employee performance appraisal

5. a. accounts payable ledger

6. a. Mixing calcium gluconate and sodium phosphate together in a syringe will cause an insoluble precipitate of calcium phosphate.

7. d. A suspension contains undissolved drug particles.

8. d. A POS system is a point-of-sale system that deducts products from inventory when they are sold.

9. d. Aspirin is contraindicated for a patient on warfarin, because it can increase bleeding of the stomach lining, thin the blood, and decrease coagulation.

10. d. all of the above

11. b. The Omnibus Budget Reconciliation Act of 1990 required pharmacists to perform drug utilization reviews, keep proper records, and counsel Medicaid patients.

12. b. A disintegrator is added to facilitate dissolution of the drug.

13. a. Most capsules are available in either hard-shell or soft-shell gelatin or some other form of soluble material.

14. b. Venlafaxine

15. d. Methyldopa is approved to treat HTN during pregnancy.

16. b. Of the available answers, clonidine is the only one used to treat hypertension and available in a patch.

17. a. Total parts = 100. Therefore 12.5 parts/100 parts $\times$ 454 grams = 56.75 grams.

18. a. Lidocaine is used to treat arrhythmias.

19. a. Of the choices, digitalis is the only drug used for atrial flutter and fibrillation.

20. b. Phytonadione produces the opposite effect as warfarin.

21. a. Safe Medical Devices Act

22. b. DEA Form 222 is used to order CII drugs.

23. d. angina pectoris

24. c. Total parts = 15.5. 1.5 parts/15.5 parts $\times$ 12 kg = 1.16 kg.

25. d. Non–potassium-sparing diuretics cause loss of potassium along with the fluid that is lost. Potassium supplements are usually given in conjunction with a drug of this nature.

26. d. Tetracycline causes the skin to be more sensitive to sunlight.

27. d. A sig code is used to facilitate order entry.

28. d. Whenever state and federal guidelines differ, always follow the guideline that is the most strict.

29. d. $\dfrac{100 \text{ mg}}{\text{ml}} = \dfrac{500 \text{ mg}}{x \text{ ml}}$

    $100x = 500$

    $x = 5 \text{ ml}$

30. c. 1 gram = 1000 mg

    $\dfrac{1000 \text{ mg}}{10 \text{ ml}} = \dfrac{600 \text{ mg}}{x}$

    $1000x = 6000$

    $x = 6 \text{ ml}$

31. d. Controlled substances can be kept under lock and key or dispersed in the regular stock in a way that deters diversion and theft.

32. b. Survanta is a natural bovine lung extract.

33. a. Consuming alcohol while using this drug will cause an antabuse-type reaction, including severe nausea and profuse vomiting.

34. d. The Kefauver-Harris amendment was passed because of birth defects due to thalidomide.

35. b. Tetracycline and tetracycline-derivative drugs should never be administered with antacids or dairy products. This medication will bind to the antacids or dairy products and simply pass through without being absorbed systemically.

36. a. Patients should always be advised to drink plenty of water when taking trimethoprim and sulfamethoxazole, to prevent crystalluria and stone formation.

37. c. Antibiotics by nature kill or inhibit microorganisms.

38. b. The lot number is needed to identify the recalled drug product.

39. c. Syringes used for oral liquid medications must not be able to accept a needle, to ensure proper administration of the liquid.

40. d. The Drug Enforcement Administration is the federal agency responsible for enforcing the CSA.

41. c. pc means after meals.

42. c. Prescriptions are not the primary records of acquisition by a pharmacy.

43. c. A broad-spectrum drug works against both gram-positive and gram-negative organisms.

44. b. 165 lb ÷ 2.2 lb/kg = 75 kg.

45. d. Fat-soluble vitamins are A, D, E, and K.

46. c. The maximum amount the patient is prescribed is 2 tabs every 4 hours, which is 12 tabs per day. 12 tabs × 14 days = 168 tablets.

47. d. A gel-cap is the only choice for masking the taste.

48. a. If the patient is to receive 1.5 mg/minute, then he or she will receive 90 mg/hr (1.5 mg × 60). The concentration of the IV is 8 mg/ml (2000 mg/250 ml).

$$\frac{8 \text{ mg}}{\text{ml}} = \frac{90 \text{ mg}}{x}$$
$$8x = 90$$
$$x = 11.25 \text{ ml; round down to } 11 \text{ ml/hr}$$

49. b. Type I diabetes is considered insulin-dependent.

50. d

51. b.
$$\frac{2 \text{ mEq}}{\text{ml}} = \frac{30 \text{ mEq}}{x}$$
$$2x = 30$$
$$x = 15 \text{ ml}$$

52. d. MAC is the maximum allowable cost.

53. d. all of the above

54. a. Class I drugs are not approved for legal use in the United States.

55. d.
$$\frac{x}{100} = \frac{150 \text{ g}}{3785}$$
$$3785x = 15,000$$
$$x = 3.96$$

56. b. Anabolic steroids are Schedule III drugs.

57. a. The Poison Prevention Packaging Act requires drugs to be dispensed in child-resistant containers unless the drug is exempt or the patient/prescriber requests otherwise.

58. c. Fosamax

59. d. Digoxin is a cardiac glycoside.

60. b. Morphine is classified as an opiate.

61. d. Oxytocin is used to induce labor contractions.

62. b. Antihypertensives manage high blood pressure.

63. b. The Prescription Drug Marketing Act prohibits the sale of drug samples.

64. d. After continued used, a patient may build up a tolerance to a drug and may require higher doses.

65. c. Dr. Jones, AJ1234563, follows the format for a valid DEA number.

66. c. Syrup of ipecac is used to induce vomiting.

67. d. The pharmacy's policies and procedures manual is the best choice for inventory procedures specific to your pharmacy.

68. c. Turnover

69. b. Hypoglycemia: hypo = low, glycemia = sugar

70. a. The law does not specifically state that the sale must be made by the pharmacist or a certified pharmacy technician.

71. b. Insulin is not derived from horse.

72. a. The patient's phone number is not required to be written on a prescription.

73. a. Patients with an allergy to penicillin are more likely to have a cross-sensitivity to cephalsporins.

74. c. 100/5000 = 0.02

75. c. NDC numbers are divided into three sections, with the first five digits indicating the manufacturer; the next four digits indicating the product name, strength, and dosage form; and the last two digits indicating the package size.

76. c. The pharmacy technician should always follow the specific policy of the pharmacy.

77. d. A 5-micron filter is the standard size for filtering particulates.

78. a. employee handbook

79. b. accounts receivable ledger

80. b. managed care
81. b
82. c. informed consent
83. a. pharmaceutical care
84. a. Class I recall has the possibility of severe complications or death.
85. d. both b and c
86. b. a wholesaler
87. b. Drug samples cannot be sold or distributed by a licensed pharmacy.
88. c. The Durham-Humphrey Amendment first distinguished between OTC and prescription drugs.
89. c. compounding
90. a. $\dfrac{3}{100} = \dfrac{x}{454}$

$100x = 1362$

$x = 13.62$ grams $\times 1000$ mg/gram $= 13,620$ mg

Practice Certification Exam III

1. d
2. a. An interface is a connection between two or more computer systems.
3. b. the process by which a nongovernmental agency or association grants recognition to an individual who has met certain predetermined qualifications specified by that agency or association
4. b. quality assurance
5. a. Sterile product preparation should be performed 6 inches from the front edge of the hood.
6. d. 1.5 gm = 1500 mg. If the concentration is 250 mg/ml, then the total volume contains 1500 mg.

$\dfrac{250 \text{ mg}}{\text{ml}} = \dfrac{1500 \text{ mg}}{x \text{ ml}}$

$250x = 1500$

$x = 6 \text{ ml}$

7. c. activities of technicians outside the workplace
8. d. The patient's telephone number is not required on a prescription label.
9. c. as many times as the prescriber indicates on the prescription within a specified time period
10. a. CI drugs have no accepted medical use in the United States.
11. c. 50 g
12. d. Add 3 + 9 + 4 = 16. Add 6 + 1 + 5 = 12 × 2 = 24. Add sums 16 + 24 = 40. Therefore, the check digit is 0.
13. b. Household cleaners must be packaged in child-proof containers.
14. a. placed under the tongue
15. d. 0.9% sodium chloride is considered isotonic.

16. d. OBRA 90 requires DURs, record keeping, and counseling
17. c. Alprazolam
18. a. Synthroid is measured in micrograms.
19. a. Legend drugs require a prescription.
20. d. Patients do not have to be paid to participate in investigational studies.
21. d. 1.5 tsp = 7.5 ml. 7.5 ml × 3 (TID) × 10 days = 225 mL
22. d. Technicians cannot dispense drug information.
23. b. Because the prescription does not specify otic or ophthalmic, the pharmacist must contact the prescriber for verification/clarification.
24. d. Tagamet and cimetidine are H_2 antagonists indicated for ulcers.
25. d. 750 mg × 2 doses per day × 7 days = 10,500 mg/1000 mg per vial = 10.5 vials. Therefore the technician needs 11 vials to prepare the order.
26. d. Final volume − diluent volume = powder volume. 50 − 34.6 = 15.4 ml.
27. d. $\dfrac{25}{100} = \dfrac{x}{480}$

$100x = 480 \times 25$

$100x = 12,000$

$x = 120$

28. b. This error code means that the patient is not enrolled in the insurance program or that the patient's name is misspelled; check for errors.
29. c. Only regular insulin can be given IV.
30. c. Deductible amounts must be met before third parties begin coverage.
31. d. Oral ampicillin suspension is not sterile; therefore, it does not need to be prepared using aseptic technique.
32. d. The ADI does not contain specifics regarding parenteral medications; it includes only trade/generic names, indications, etc.
33. d. all of the above
34. b. Notify the pharmacist that the patient has orders for two drugs of the same class.
35. c. Discreetly notify the pharmacist so that the appropriate action may be taken.
36. d. Etoposide is a chemotherapy drug, so it should not be mixed in a horizontal hood, but in a vertical hood or biological safety cabinet.
37. b. Because technicians cannot provide drug information, the technician should inform the pharmacist that the mother would like help choosing a non-prescription product.

38. c. Patient package inserts are required with oral inhalers.

39. a. Notify the pharmacist if the patient is also buying aspirin; there is an interaction between these medications, and the patient should not take the medications together.

40. c. A technician can answer this question because it does not involve professional judgment or drug information.

41. b. A strength is needed to fill the prescription, so the technician should alert the pharmacist to the problem.

42. d. All the choices could contribute to a medication error. Failure to rotate stock could result in dispensing an expired or short-date drug; preparing more than one prescription at a time could result in the wrong medication going to the wrong patient; and not reading the label could result in the wrong drug or strength being used.

43. b. Trailing zeros (7.0 mg) should not be used because if the decimal point is not clear, the amount could be mistaken for 70 mg, not 7 mg.

44. d. all of the above

45. c. Explain the situation to the pharmacist, correct the error, document the error per procedure, and have the patient return to the pharmacy for the correct prescription.

46. c. Diazepam is a CIV drug and is not ordered on Form 222.

47. c. Unit-dose medications are not patient-specific; therefore, patient information is not printed directly on the drug label.

48. a. A technician should never call a prescriber for clarification on an abbreviation.

49. d. Refer the question to the pharmacist, because technicians cannot dispense drug information.

50. a. o.u. = both eyes.

51. d. 30 cc = 30 ml = 2 Tbsp

52. a. Oral polio vaccine is frozen for long-term storage.

53. d. When only a month and year are given in an expiration date, the drug is usable until the last day of that month.

54. b. U-100 means 100 units/ml. Therfore, 35 units = 0.35 ml.

55. d. Vinblastine is a chemotherapy drug.

56. d. Prescribers can give CIII drugs a maximum of five refills that must be used within six months after date of issuance.

57. b. cyclophosphamide

58. d. aseptic technique

59. c. carbamazepine

60. d. all of the above

61. d. Triazolam is a hypnotic used to induce sleep.

62. a. a.u. = both ears, therefore an otic suspension should be dispensed.

63. d. 2000 ml ÷ 10 hr = 200 ml/hr

64. c. 100 ÷ 1000 = 0.1

65. b. The full quantity of the original prescription is for a 12-month supply (3 months with 3 refills). Therefore, if 1 month's worth is dispensed, the patient will get 11 refills for a 12-month supply.

66. c. Ask the patient the type of allergic reaction experienced, note the patient's response, and alert the pharmacist so the pharmacist can question the patient regarding the reaction.

67. b. If a prescription is marked (according to state law) that no substitutions are allowed, then a trade name must be dispensed unless the prescriber is contacted to okay a substitution.

68. c. 1 tbsp = 15 ml; 360 ml/15 ml per tbsp = 24 tbsp

69. b. 1 fluid ounce = 30 ml; 3 × 30 = 90

70. d. 1 mg = 1000 mcg; a 950-mcg dose = 0.95 mg.

$$\frac{0.05 \text{ mg}}{\text{ml}} = \frac{0.95 \text{ mg}}{x}$$
$$0.5x = 0.95$$
$$x = 1.9$$

71. b. If the patient wants the insurance to pay the maximum amount, then the generic drug must be dispensed.

72. d. The last step in filling a new prescription is RPh counseling.

73. d. All drug interaction messaging should be directed to the pharmacist.

74. d. 500 mg × 4 (qid) × 7 = 14,000 mg; 14,000 mg/250-mg tablets = 56 tablets.

75. a. $\frac{125 \text{ mg}}{5 \text{ ml}} = \frac{250 \text{ mg}}{x \text{ ml}}$

$$125x = 1250$$
$$x = 10 \text{ ml}$$

10 ml × 3 (tid) × 10 days = 300 mL

76. d. Alert the pharmacist about any drug interaction messages.

77. c. Cefazolin is an antibiotic.

78. d. The physician's DEA number is required on all controlled-substance prescriptions, but not on the prescription container labels.

79. b. The tip and plunger must remain sterile.

80. d. Vertical flow hoods provide the best preparer protection, because contaminated air is not blown at the operator.

81. a. Amphotericin B must be protected from light. IV bags are covered with amber bags.

82. c. Tobramycin injection does not have to be refrigerated. IVs compounded with the injection should be refrigerated.

83. a. Sepsis is a severe infection in the body and is not normally treated at home.

84. c. Cefotaxime is a cephalosporin antibiotic, not chemotherapy or hazardous

85. d. Pancrease is not a laxative.

86. a. Tobramycin is available as an injection, topical cream, and ophthalmic solution.

87. d. Ibuprofen is available only in oral dosage forms.

88. b. $\dfrac{80 \text{ mg}}{2 \text{ ml}} = \dfrac{130 \text{ mg}}{x \text{ ml}}$

$$80x = 130$$
$$x = 3.25 \text{ ml}$$

89. b. $\dfrac{1000 \text{ ml}}{480 \text{ min}} = \dfrac{10 \text{ gtt}}{\text{ml}} = 20.8 \text{ gtt/min}$

Round up to 21 gtt/min.

90. c. Federal law does not allow refills on CII drugs.

Practice Certification Exam IV

1. b. Zovirax

2. d. In clinical pharmacy, the pharmacist uses his or her drug information expertise to enhance and optimize patient care and outcomes.

3. d. Each state has its own state board of pharmacy, which creates and enforces all pharmacy licensing and laws in that state.

4. d. The active ingredient causes the desired effect.

5. d. Suspensions and emulsions contain particles that are not dissolved, so they are considered suspensions.

6. d. The DEA Form 222 has 10 lines; therefore, a maximum of 10 different drugs could be ordered on one form.

7. d

8. c. Patient profiles should always be updated with correct information.

9. c. Always follow the return policies of your pharmacy.

10. a. *Remington's Pharmaceutical Sciences* is the go-to source for information on compounding medications.

11. d. When patients take their medication as directed, they are complying with the prescription.

12. d. The five rights of medication administration are the right route, the right dose, the right medication, the right patient, and the right time.

13. b. The FDA regulates GMPs.

14. a. Hiring practices for the organization may not be found in the pharmacy's P&P manual, but in the organization's P&P manual.

15. d. 0.75 gm = 750 mg; therefore, the patient needs 15 ml or 1 tablespoon.

16. d. Vitamin B-1 is thiamine.

17. c. 1000 mcg = 1 mg; therefore the patient is to receive 1 mg per minute. 1 mg × 60 minutes = 60 mg per hour. The concentration of the IV is 2 mg/ml (500 mg/250 ml), so the IV rate is 30 mg/ml.

18. b. A patient's insurance coverage should not affect the drug dosage that the physician prescribes.

19. c. Because the active ingredients in a liquid are already dissolved, they will deteriorate faster than those that have to dissolve in the body.

20. b. Batch repackaging involves repackaging large amounts for general use in the pharmacy. Extemporaneous repackaging is repackaging a drug for a specific patient or order.

21. c. 8 fl oz = 240 ml

$$70x = 50 \times 240$$
$$70x = 12,000$$
$$x = 171.4 \text{ ml}$$

22. c. Efudex is a topical chemotherapy drug used to treat solar keratoses.

23. d. Using the NDC will ensure that the correct drug is pulled from the shelf and used to fill the prescription.

24. b. Pharmacies are required to have a Class A prescription balance.

25. b. A compounding slab is used to mix topical medications.

26. c. A "refill too soon" message indicates that the days' supply entered in the computer does not match how the patient is using the drug. Either the patient is using the drug incorrectly or the pharmacy entered the days' supply incorrectly.

27. c. Prn means as needed, therefore a prn drug is given only under specific circumstances and is not scheduled around the clock.

28. b. Isotretinoin is used to treat acne; if it is taken by a pregnant woman, it can cause birth defects or miscarriage.

29. c. The ScriptPro is used to fill retail prescriptions; the Automix is used to compound TPNs; and the Pyxis and Omnicell are automated medication dispensing devices used in hospital settings.

30. d

31. c. Technicians must always refer drug information or counseling questions to the pharmacist.

32. b. 4 oz = 120 ml. A 3:1 ratio has a total of 4 parts. If you divide 120 ml by 4 parts, you get 30 ml for each part. Therefore: 3 × 30 ml = 90 and 1 × 30 ml = 30 ml.

33. c. $1.5^2 \, m^2 \times 20 \, mg/m^2 = 30.4$ mg per day

$$\frac{50 \, mg}{50 \, ml} = \frac{30.4 \, mg}{x \, ml}$$

$$50x = 1520$$

$$x = 30.4 \, ml$$

34. b. $\dfrac{10 \, mg}{ml} = \dfrac{40 \, mg}{x \, ml}$

$$10x = 40$$

$$x = 4 \, ml \text{ for each dose}$$

4 ml per dose $\times$ 3 doses per day (q8h) = 12 ml total. Therefore, you need to send 2 mdv.

35. c. 2000 ml $\div$ 24 hr = 83.3 ml/hr. Round down to 83 ml/hr.

36. c. $\dfrac{250 \, mg}{5 \, ml} = \dfrac{375 \, mg}{x \, ml}$

$$250x = 375(5)$$

$$250x = 1875$$

$$x = 7.5 \, ml = 1½ \, tsp$$

37. b. Rifampin will cause discoloration of the urine and feces.

38. b. U-100 means 100 units per milliliter.

39. d. Percodan contains aspirin, so it should not be taken because of the interaction between warfarin and aspirin.

40. d. Antibiotics are often considered an "automatic stop order," which means that the pharmacy will automatically stop filling the order after a predetermined period of time unless the doctor renews or reorders the medication. This will prevent patients from taking antibiotics for extended periods of time, which in turn could cause drug resistance.

41. c. $100 \div 10,000 = 0.01$

42. d. During medication delivery rounds, or simply "rounds," the technician picks up new orders and drops off orders that have been filled.

43. a. The IV route has the fastest onset of action, because the drug is injected directly into the bloodstream.

44. b. Unit-dose drug packages are not specific to any one patient. Therefore the patient's name is not on the drug label.

45. c. Drugs that require patient package inserts (PPIs) must include them with each prescription or refill.

46. d. $42.10 \div 100 = $0.421 for each tablet

$0.421 \times 60 tablets = $25.26 for 60 tabs

$25.25 + (25.25 \times 0.25) = $31.575; rounded to the nearest penny = $31.58

47. d

48. a. 0.5% means 0.5 gm per 100 gm.

$$\frac{0.5 \, gm}{100 \, mg} = \frac{x \, gm}{120 \, gm}$$

$$100x = 60$$

$$x = 0.6 \, gm$$

49. b. $\dfrac{30 \, mg}{5 \, ml} = \dfrac{38.4 \, mg}{x \, ml}$

$$30x = 192$$

$$x = 6.4 \, ml$$

50. d. 40 lb $\div$ 2.2 kg/lb = 18.18 kg

18.18 kg $\times$ 30 mg/kg/day = 545.4 mg/day

545.4 mg/day $\div$ 2 divided doses = 272.7 mg/dose, rounded to 273 mg

51. d. 10 gm = 10,000 mg

10,000 mg $\div$ 125 mg/dose = 80 doses

52. a. The gauge refers to the diameter of the needle's shaft. The lumen refers to the inner diameter of the needle.

53. d. The IDC-9 code is the code set for diagnosis required by HIPAA standards.

54. c. 20 mg $\times$ 2 caps per dose $\times$ 2 doses per day = 80 mg per day

55. c. $\dfrac{1 \, mg}{ml} = \dfrac{x \, mg}{100 \, ml}$

$x = 100$; therefore, 100 mg is needed to prepare 100 ml of a 1-mg/ml solution.

$$\frac{10 \, mg}{tab} = \frac{100 \, mg}{x \, tab}$$

$$10x = 100$$

$$x = 10 \, tabs$$

56. c. Cyclosphosphamide is a chemotherapy drug, and a chemo spill kit is required to be near anyone who prepares or administers chemo drugs.

57. d

58. b. Nitroglycerin is required to be dispensed in its original glass container to maintain its potency.

59. d. % strength = # of grams of active ingredient per 100 gm of product. 250 mg = 0.25 gm; therefore

$$\frac{0.25 \, gm}{30 \, gm} = \frac{x \, gm}{100 \, gm}$$

$$30x = 25$$

$$x = 0.8333$$

$x = 0.8333$ gm are in 100 gm of product; therefore the percent strength is 0.83%.

60. d. All unused investigational drugs should be returned to the manufacturer per guidelines.

61. c. The generic name for Pamelor is nortriptyline.

62. a. Perpetual inventory maintains a running total of all inventory. Therfore, the pharmacy must document all sales and purchases as they occur.

63. b. NDC numbers are divided into three sections, with the first five digits indicating the manufacturer; the next four digits indicating the product name, strength, and dosage form; and the last two digits indicating the package size.

64. c. As drugs are ordered and placed into inventory, the drugs with the shortest expiration date should be moved to the front of the shelf to ensure that those drugs are used first.

65. b. A hospital formulary is a listing of all approved drugs used in the institution.

66. c. Acetaminophen with codeine is a Schedule III drug.

67. d. A purchase order shows the technician what drugs have been ordered.

68. c. Inventory turnover indicates how often the pharmacy uses its inventory.

69. c. When only a month and year are indicated on an expiration date, the drug is usable until the last day of that month.

70. c. Meperidine is a CII drug, and all CIIs are ordered on a DEA Form 222.

71. b. Actos is an oral antidiabetic drug.

72. b. A PAR level indicates the minimum level to be kept on the shelf. If the level falls below the PAR level, then the technician orders enough drug to bring the quantity up to the PAR level.

73. c. The *Physician's Desk Reference* contains a compilation of manufacturers' package inserts.

74. b. Paxil is indicated for the treatment of major depressive episode.

75. d. If the patient has already been taking the medication, the best choice is to find the patient a pharmacy that stocks the drug.

76. c. Insurance claim errors decrease the payments received by the pharmacy.

77. b. Refrigeration temperature range is $2-8°C$ or $36-46°F$.

78. c. If possible, always document any damage or missing boxes before the delivery person leaves the pharmacy.

79. a. Class I recalls have the potential for serious harm or death to the patient.

80. d. The Occupational Safety and Health Administration requires MSDSs.

81. d. Diazepam is not exempt. Oral inhalers, nitroglycerin sl tabs and all hospital unit dose medications are exempt.

82. b. If a refill section is left blank, then the pharmacy must not give any refills.

83. c. The Omnibus Budget Reconciliation Act requires pharmacists to counsel Medicaid patients.

84. d. Any person (pharmacist or tech) who signs a DEA Form 222 must have the power to do so.

85. b. At a minimum, compounding equipment must be cleaned at least once daily, usually before use.

Equipment should also be cleaned after it is used and anytime it is contaminated.

86. c. Pharmaceutical scales and balances should be certified for accuracy at least yearly.

87. d. All health care providers (doctors, pharmacists, pharmacy technicians), health plans (insurance company), and health care clearing houses are considered covered entities.

88. c. ScriptPro is used in retail Pharmacies; Pyxis, Omnicell, and AcuDose are used in institutional settings.

89. d. Policies and procedures manuals contain all the pharmacy's best practices.

90. c

Practice Certification Exam V

1. a. Co-payment is a set amount that the patient pays for each prescription.

2. c. Drugs are not necessarily used for life-sustaining or supporting efforts.

3. c. A five-drawer filing system is not allowed.

4. a. There is no particular pH level that an IV should have, although infusion of isotonic IVs is easier on the patient and causes fewer complications.

5. b. 4 tabs daily $\times$ 2 days = 8 tabs
   3 tabs daily $\times$ 2 days = 6 tabs
   1 tab BID $\times$ 2 days = 4 tabs
   ½ tab BID $\times$ 2 days = 2 tabs
   ½ tab daily $\times$ 2 days = 1 tab
   Total = 21 tabs

6. a. 1000 ml/480 min $\times$ 20 gtt/ml = 41.6; round up to 42 gtt/min.

7. c. The patient's phone number is not required on the prescription label. All other information is required.

8. a. Sterilizing filters are 0.2 microns or smaller in size.

9. d. 150 ml ÷ 50 ml/hr = 3 hr

10. a. Laminar airflow hoods are designed to provide an ultraclean, almost sterile environment for IV preparation.

11. b. Proper aseptic technique minimizes the chance of contaminating sterile products.

12. a. Reorder points indicate the maximum and minimum amounts of inventory to be kept.

13. b. Unlike a side effect, an adverse effect is usually severe in nature and is not expected.

14. b. Prescriptions in the institutional setting are called medication orders, physician's orders, doctor's orders, drug orders, or orders.

15. b. MSDSs contain information on what to do if you have an accident with the substance on the sheet.

16. a. 0.5 kg × 1000 g/kg = 500 g

    25 mg × 1 g/1000 g = 0.025 g

    10 g + 500 g + 0.025 g = 510.025 g

17. c. Drugs destroyed in the liver during the first-pass effect are not absorbed into the body

18. c. The CSA classified controlled substances into one of five schedules based on abuse potential.

19. c. PR stands for per rectum or rectally

20. c. Only one item may be ordered per line on DEA Form 222.

21. c. U&C stands for usual and customary.

22. b. Continuous infusions run at a slow constant rate over a long period of time.

23. a. DEA Form 222 is used to order CII medications.

24. c. Intermittent infusions are small volumes given over short periods of time. IVPBs are a type of intermittent infusion.

25. d. 1.17 kg × 1000 g/kg = 1170 g

    260 mg × 1 g/1000 mg = 0.26 g

    1170 + 1.59 + 0.26 = 1171.85 g

26. d. All of these containers are considered for one time usage.

27. d. Patient confidentiality is mandated by the federal law HIPAA.

28. c. Sig means directions for use.

29. c. Phosphate should be added first, then all other additives should be added; the TPN should be mixed in between additions. Add any calcium last, before any drug with color.

30. b. A point-of-sale (POS) system maintains a continuous record of all inventory items purchased and sold.

31. b. 2 kg = 2000 gm = 2,000,000 mg. Therefore, 2,000,000 mg ÷ 325 mg = 6153.8 tablets can be made from the acetaminophen. 5 gm = 5000 mg. Therefore, 5000 mg ÷ 2 mg = 2500 tablets can be made from the chlorpheniramine.

32. b. Normal saline (0.9% sodium chloride) is isotonic.

33. d. 1 capsules are the smallest in size. The larger the capsule number, the smaller the capsule size.

34. d. GERD is gastroesophogeal reflux disease, and esomeprazole is used to tread GERD.

35. d. Nitroglycerin is good for only approximately six months after the glass bottle is opened, even if the medication is still within the manufacturer's expiration date.

36. c. Expiration dates with the month and year indicate that the drug is good until the last day of the month.

37. d. Because the patient is administering the IV at home, the directions must be transcribed out for the patient.

38. c. Sedatives and hypnotics are Schedule IV controlled substances.

39. a. $\dfrac{250 \text{ mg}}{x \text{ ml}} = \dfrac{12.5 \text{ mg}}{\text{ml}}$

    $12.5x = 250$

    $x = 20$ ml

40. a. 3500 ml of Dextrose 10% can be made from 500 ml of Dextrose 70%.

41. c. Fluorouracil is a chemotherapy drug.

42. d. 25,000 units ÷ 500 ml = 50 units/ml

43. a. The *Handbook of Injectable Drugs* is the go-to guide for parenteral medications.

44. d. Pharmacy techs are involved in all of the processes.

45. d. Checking refrigerator temps are all of the above.

46. a. No drugs can be dispensed by a pharmacy technician without a pharmacist's approval.

47. d. It is within a technician's scope of duty to retrieve lab data for the pharmacist to use in making clinical judgments on patient care. As long as the technician is not making any judgments on the patient's care.

48. a. If a generic substitution is made, the drugs must have the same active ingredient and cause the same effect on the body.

49. d. USP 797 requires that sterile alcohol and sterile water be used.

50. d. All the statements are true.

51. d. Technicians should not call a doctor to discuss drug therapy.

52. d. Technicians cannot counsel, but they can instruct someone to call poison control.

53. d. A package insert is prepared by the manufacturer and is intended for the clinician.

54. a. Always notify the pharmacist if you see a potential drug interaction such as between cisapride and fluconazole.

55. d. ADI provides all the above information.

56. b. MSDSs do not give specific antidote dosing.

57. d. Oral inhalers usually are not taken with food.

58. b. $6.80 − (6.80 × 40%) = $4.08

59. c. The oral route is the easiest and least complicated ROA.

60. b. A troche is also called a lozenge.

61. d. Pastilles are sucked in the mouth.

62. b. Extended-release medications are designed to release medication over longer periods of time, therefore reducing the frequency of doses.

63. b. PR = rectally

64. d. Hydromorphone is a CII drug.

65. d. $\dfrac{24 \text{ mEq}}{x \text{ ml}} = \dfrac{08 \text{ mEq}}{\text{ml}}$

$$0.8x = 24$$
$$x = 30 \text{ ml}$$

66. d. Vitamin K is necessary for proper blood coagulation.

67. d. Technicians are responsible for all the duties in home care.

68. c. This type of reimbursement is called capitation.

69. d. All the above types of data can be collected by the technician at the in window.

70. c. 32.5 ml of a 10 mg/5 ml drug will deliver a dose of 65 mg.

71. d. All the above are examples of quality control.

72. b. A patient's deductable must be met before an insurance company will begin to pay additional benefits or expenses.

73. d. Gowns, gloves, and masks should be worn when preparing chemotherapy or hazardous drugs.

74. b. 1 tab × 2 doses per day × 10 days = 20 tabs

75. d. Techs are only allowed to fill med carts and are generally not allowed to perform any of the other duties.

76. d. The Joint Commission requires the separation of dosage forms for safety reasons.

77. b. Controlled substances usually have an automatic stop order, which means the pharmacy will stop filling the order after a predetermined period of time unless the doctor renews the order.

78. c. 1 tbsp = 15 ml

15 ml × 32 = 480 ml

79. d. For extended stability, amphotericin should be mixed in D5W.

80. d. Baxa is a pharmaceutical company, not an automated dispensing system.

81. c. Never recap needles before disposal.

82. a. Phentermine is indicated for the short-term use in weight reduction along with exercise and diet.

83. c. The prescriber's signature is required on the original prescription, but it is not on the prescription label.

84. a. Erythromycin 2% solution is a topical solution.

85. b. Cimetidine is an H_2 antagonist and is not generally found on a crash cart.

86. b. Line 2 has the first error. The balance should be 45 not 44.

87. b. Only a signature can prove that a patient picked up a prescription.

88. d. 1 L = 1000 mL

1000 mL ÷ 125 mL/hr = 8 hr

Each 1-L bag will last 8 hours, so three 1-L bags are needed for a 24-hour supply.

89. b. Proper hand washing is the most basic and effective way for a technician to prevent contamination.

90. d. Etodolac is indicated for osteoarthritis and rheumatoid arthritis.

Math Practice Test I

1. b. 0.25% × x ml = 0.1% × 500 ml

$$0.25x = 50$$
$$x = 200 \text{ ml}$$

2. b. 100 tabs ÷ 5 tabs per day = 20-day supply

3. d. $\dfrac{2 \text{ mg}}{5 \text{ ml}} = \dfrac{3 \text{ mg}}{x \text{ ml}}$

$$2x = 15$$
$$x = 7.5 \text{ ml per dose}$$

7.5 ml per dose × 3 doses per day (TID) × 14 days = 315 ml

4. c. 1% × x gm = 0.5% × 60 gm

$$x = 30 \text{ gm}$$

5. a. $10.23 ÷ 100 tabs = $0.1023 per tab

$0.1023 × 90 tabs = $9.207

$9.207 + (9.207 × 32%) = $12.15324 + 4.50
= 16.65324; round to $16.65

6. b. 70% × x ml = 25% × 1000 ml

$$70x = 25{,}000$$
$$x = 357.14; \text{ round to } 357 \text{ ml}$$

7. d. 1 tbsp = 15 ml

4350 ÷ 15 = 290

8. d. 1 tsp = 5 ml

12.5 ÷ 5 = 2.5

9. b. 35,000 units/1000 ml = 35 units/ml

5 units/ml × 20 ml/hr = 700 units/hr

10. d. 1 tab × 4 doses per day × 90 days = 360 tabs

11. c. 100 caps ÷ 4 caps per day = 25-day supply

12. b. 26.4 lb ÷ 2.2 lb/kg = 12 kg

12 kg × 30 mg per day = 360 mg per day

360 mg ÷ 3 doses per day = 120 mg per dose

$$\dfrac{125 \text{ mg}}{5 \text{ ml}} = \dfrac{120 \text{ mg}}{x \text{ ml}}$$

$$125x = 600$$
$$x = 4.8 \text{ ml}$$

13. d. ½ NS = 0.45% sodium chloride

Percent strength = # grams per 100 ml

$$\dfrac{0.45 \text{ gm}}{100 \text{ ml}} = \dfrac{x \text{ gm}}{500 \text{ ml}}$$

$$100x = 225$$
$$x = 2.25 \text{ g}$$

14. a. Powder volume = final volume − diluent volume. After reconstitution, if 10 ml has 1 gm of drug, then the total volume of the vial is 20 ml, because it is a 2-gm vial.

$x = 20$ ml $− 15.5$

$x = 4.5$ ml

15. c. If the patient is receiving 1400 units per hour, then you need to calculate how many milliliters contain 1400 units.

Concentration: 40,000 units ÷ 1000 ml
= 40 units/ml

$$\frac{40 \text{ units}}{\text{ml}} = \frac{1400 \text{ units}}{x \text{ ml}}$$

$40x = 1400$

$x = 35$ ml

Therefore the IV will run at 35 ml/hr.

16. c. 48 lb ÷ 2.2 lb/kg = 21.82 kg

21.82 kg × 20 mg/kg = 436.4 mg per day

436.4 mg ÷ 3 doses per day = 145.47 mg

$$\frac{187 \text{ mg}}{5 \text{ ml}} = \frac{145.47 \text{ mg}}{x \text{ ml}}$$

$187x = 727.35$

$x = 3.88$; round to 3.9 ml

17. d. $$\frac{70 \text{ gm}}{100 \text{ ml}} = \frac{x \text{ gm}}{80 \text{ ml}}$$

$100x = 5600$

$x = 56$ gm $× 1000 = 56,000$ mg

18. b. 3 gm × 9 doses = 27 grams are needed.

27 gm ÷ 10 gm/vial = 2.7 vials, which means you need 3 vials.

19. c. Percent strength = gm per 100. Therefore, if you 100 ml of 30%, you have 30 gm of active drug.

20. b. 3785 ml/gal × 2.5 gal = 9462.5 ml

$$\frac{45.6 \text{ gm}}{100 \text{ ml}} = \frac{x \text{ gm}}{9462.5 \text{ ml}}$$

$10x = 431,490$

$x = 4314.9$ gm

21. c. $23.40 ÷ 100 = 0.234 per cap × 60 caps
= $14.04

$14.04 + (14.04 × 40%) = 19.656 = $19.66

22. c. 0.5 gm = 500 mg

$$\frac{250 \text{ mg}}{5 \text{ ml}} = \frac{500 \text{ mg}}{x \text{ ml}}$$

$250x = 2500$

$x = 10$ ml

23. c. $$\frac{258 \text{ ml}}{946 \text{ ml}} = \frac{x \text{ ml}}{100 \text{ ml}}$$

$946x = 25,800$

$x = 27.3$ ml

If there are 27.27 ml of drug in 100 ml, then the percentage is 27.3%.

24. d. $$\frac{56 \text{ gm}}{473 \text{ ml}} = \frac{x \text{ gm}}{100 \text{ ml}}$$

$473x = 5600$

$x = 11.8$ gm

If there are 11.8 gm of drug in 100 ml, then the percentage is 11.8%.

25. c. IV conc = 40,000 units/1000 ml = 40 units/ml

$$\frac{40 \text{ units}}{\text{ml}} = \frac{2000 \text{ units}}{x \text{ ml}}$$

$40x = 2000$

$x = 50$ ml

Therefore the IV rate is 50 ml/hr. Now 50 ml/60 min × 15 gtt/ml = 12.5, rounded to 13 gtt/min.

26. c. 100 ÷ 10,000 = 0.01

27. b. 1 gr = 65 mg

325 mg ÷ 65 mg/gr = 5 gr

28. c. 100 ÷ 5 = 20; therefore the ratio is 1:20.

29. d. $$\frac{10 \text{ mg}}{5 \text{ ml}} = \frac{50 \text{ mg}}{x \text{ ml}}$$

$10x = 250$

$x = 25$ ml

30. d. Sterile water contains 0% of sorbitol.

70		25
	25	
0		45

Total

Parts 70

$$\frac{25}{70} × 500 \text{ ml} = 178.57 \text{ ml of 70%}$$

$$\frac{45}{70} × 500 \text{ ml} = 321.4 \text{ ml of sterile water}$$

Math Practice Test II

1. d. 12.5 × x ml = 10 × 500 ml

$12.5x = 50,000$

$x = 400$ ml

2. d. 60 tabs ÷ 1.5 tabs per day = 40-day supply

3. b. $$\frac{2 \text{ mg}}{5 \text{ ml}} = \frac{0.5 \text{ mg}}{x \text{ ml}}$$

$2x = 2.5$

$x = 1.25$ ml per dose

1.25 ml per dose × 3 doses per day (TID) × 30 days = 112.5 ml

4. c. 2.5% × x gm = 0.25% × 120 gm

$x = 12$ gm

5. a. $23.80 ÷ 100 tabs = $0.238 per tab

$0.238 × 30 tabs = $7.14

$7.14 + (7.14 × 40%) = 9.996 + 6.50 = 16.496, rounded to $16.50

6. a. 70% × x ml = 10% × 500 ml

$70x = 5000$

$x = 71.428$, rounded to 71 ml

7. c. 500 mg × 1.3 m^2 = 650 mg per day

650 mg ÷ 2 doses per day = 325 mg per dose

8. d. 1 tsp = 5 ml

$25 ÷ 5 = 5$

9. a. 35,000 units/1000 ml = 35 units/ml

35 units/ml × 10 ml/hr = 350 units/hr

10. c. 2 tabs × 4 doses per day × 30 days = 240 tabs

11. d. 90 caps ÷ 2 caps per day = 45-day supply

12. b. 22 kg = 48.4 lbs

(48.4 lbs × 200 mg)/150 = 64.5 mg

13. d. NS = 0.9% sodium chloride. Percent strength = # grams per 100 ml; therefore

$$\frac{0.9 \text{ gm}}{100 \text{ ml}} = \frac{x \text{ gm}}{1000 \text{ ml}}$$

$100x = 900$

$x = 9$ gm

14. b. Powder volume = final volume − diluent volume

$x = 10$ ml − 9.5

$x = 0.5$ ml

15. d. If the patient is receiving 2100 units per hour, you need to calculate how many milliliters contains 2100 units.

Concentration = 30,000 units ÷ 1000 ml = 30 units/ml

$$\frac{30 \text{ units}}{\text{ml}} = \frac{2100 \text{ units}}{x \text{ ml}}$$

$30x = 2100$

$x = 70$ ml

Therefore, the IV will run at 70 ml/hr.

16. b. $\dfrac{35 × 250}{150} = 58.3$

17. c. $\dfrac{5 \text{ gm}}{100 \text{ ml}} = \dfrac{x \text{ gm}}{2500 \text{ ml}}$

$100x = 12,500$

$x = 125$ gm

18. b. 2 gm × 2 doses per day × 7 days = 28 grams needed

28 gm ÷ 10 gm/vial = 2.8 vials

Therefore, you need 3 vials.

19. d. Percent strength = gm per 100. Therefore, if you 100 ml of 70%, you have 70 gm of active drug.

20. c. $\dfrac{20 \text{ gm}}{100 \text{ ml}} = \dfrac{x \text{ gm}}{500 \text{ ml}}$

$100x = 10,000$

$x = 100$ gm

21. d. $3.40 ÷ 100 = 0.034 per cap × 30 caps = $1.02

$1.02 + (1.02 × 36%) = 1.3872 + $8.00 = 9.3872 = $9.39

22. b. $\dfrac{500,000 \text{ units}}{\text{ml}} = \dfrac{250,000 \text{ units}}{x \text{ ml}}$

$500,000x = 250,000$

$x = 0.5$ ml

23. b. $\dfrac{30 \text{ ml}}{120 \text{ ml}} = \dfrac{x \text{ ml}}{100 \text{ ml}}$

$120x = 3000$

$x = 25$ ml

If there are 25 ml of drug in 100 ml, the percentage is 25%.

24. d. $\dfrac{30 \text{ gm}}{480 \text{ ml}} = \dfrac{x \text{ gm}}{100 \text{ ml}}$

$480x = 3000$

$x = 6.25$ gm

If there are 6.25 gm of drug in 100 ml, the percentage is 6.25%.

25. b. IV concentration = 20,000 units/1000 ml = 20 units/ml

$$\frac{20 \text{ units}}{\text{ml}} = \frac{2500 \text{ units}}{x \text{ ml}}$$

$20x = 2500$

$x = 125$ ml

Therefore, the IV rate is 125 ml/hr.

125 ml/60 min × 10 gtt/ml = 20.8, rounded to 21 gtt/min

26. c. 200 ÷ 20,000 = 0.01

27. b. 1 mg = 1000 mcg

5 mg × 1000 mcg/mg = 5000 mcg

28. c. $\dfrac{500,000 \text{ units}}{\text{ml}} = \dfrac{20,000,000 \text{ units}}{x \text{ ml}}$

$500,000x = 20,000,000$

$x = 40$ ml

29. b. $\dfrac{10 \text{ mg}}{\text{ml}} = \dfrac{35 \text{ mg}}{x \text{ ml}}$

$10x = 35$

$x = 3.5$ ml

30. d. Sterile water contains 0% sorbitol.

```
70  |      10
    |  10  |
----+------+----
0   |      60
```

    Total
    Parts 70

$$\frac{10}{70} \times 500 \text{ ml} = 71.4 \text{ ml of } 70\%$$

$$\frac{60}{70} \times 500 \text{ ml} = 428.6 \text{ ml of sterile water}$$

Math Practice Test III

1. c. 75 mg × 4 doses per day = 300 mg

    $$\frac{50 \text{ mg}}{\text{ml}} = \frac{300 \text{ mg}}{x \text{ ml}}$$

    $$50x = 300$$

    $$x = 6 \text{ ml}$$

    Therefore, 6 ml are needed for the day; if each vial contains 2 ml, you need 3 vials.

2. b. 2 caps per dose × 3 doses per day × 10 days = 60 caps

3. c. $$\frac{50 \text{ mg}}{5 \text{ ml}} = \frac{30 \text{ mg}}{x \text{ ml}}$$

    $$50x = 150$$

    $$x = 3 \text{ ml per dose}$$

4. b. 0.5% × x gm = 0.0.25% × 120 gm

    $$x = 6 \text{ gm}$$

5. d. $142.50 ÷ 1000 tabs = $0.1425 per tab

    $0.1425 × 90 tabs = $12.825

    $12.825 + (12.825 × 40%) = 17.955 + 10.50 = 28.455, rounded to $28.46

6. b. 50% × x ml = 10% × 2000 ml

    $$50x = 20,000$$

    $$x = 400 \text{ ml}$$

7. d. $65.30 ÷ 100 caps = 0.653 per cap

    0.653 × 30 caps = $19.59 (cost for 30 caps)

    $19.59 × 30% = 5.877 = $5.88 (markup)

    $19.59 (cost) + $5.88 (markup) = $25.47 (selling price)

8. c. 1 tbsp = 15 ml

    450 ÷ 15 = 30

9. d. 40,000 units/500 ml = 80 units/ml

    80 units/ml × 16 ml/hr = 1280 units/hr

10. b. 1 tab × 2 doses per day × 90 days = 180 tabs

11. c. 60 tabs ÷ 4 tabs per day = 15-day supply

12. d. (6 × 250 mg)/(6 + 12) = 83.3 mg

13. d. ½ NS = 0.45% sodium chloride. Percent strength = # grams per 100 ml; therefore,

    $$\frac{0.45 \text{ mg}}{100 \text{ ml}} = \frac{x \text{ gm}}{2000 \text{ ml}}$$

    $$100x = 900$$

    $$x = 9 \text{ gm}$$

14. a. Powder volume = final volume − diluent volume

    $$\frac{100 \text{ mg}}{\text{ml}} = \frac{1000 \text{ mg}}{\text{ml}}$$

    $$100x = 1000$$

    $$x = 10 \text{ ml}$$

    If the concentration is 100 mg/ml and you have a vial of 1 gm (1000 mg), the final volume is 10 ml.

    $$x = 10 \text{ ml} - 8.5$$

    $$x = 1.5 \text{ ml}$$

15. d. If the patient is receiving 1400 units per hour, you need to calculate how many milliliters contain 1400 units.

    Concentration = 20,000 units ÷ 1000 ml = 20 units/ml

    $$\frac{20 \text{ units}}{\text{ml}} = \frac{1400 \text{ units}}{x \text{ ml}}$$

    $$20x = 1400$$

    $$x = 70 \text{ ml}$$

    The IV will run at 70 ml/hr.

16. a. 20 kg × 2.2 lb/kg = 44 lb

    $$\frac{44 \times 50}{150} = 14.666, \text{ rounded to } 14.7$$

17. d. $$\frac{0.45 \text{ gm}}{100 \text{ ml}} = \frac{x \text{ gm}}{1000 \text{ ml}}$$

    $$100x = 450$$

    $$x = 9 \text{ gm}$$

18. d. 500 mg × 100 doses = 50,000 mg

    50,000 ÷ 1000 mg/gm = 50 gm needed

    50 gm ÷ 10 gm/vial = 5 vials

19. a. Percent strength = gm per 100. Therefore, if you 100 ml of 20%, you have 20 gm of active drug.

20. c. $$\frac{25 \text{ gm}}{100 \text{ ml}} = \frac{x \text{ gm}}{2000 \text{ ml}}$$

    $$100x = 50,000$$

    $$x = 500 \text{ gm}$$

21. b. $69.87 ÷ 500 = 0.13974 per cap × 40 caps = $5.5896

    $5.5896 + (5.5896 × 16.2%) = 6.4951 + $15.30 = 21.7951 = $21.80

22. d. $$\frac{500,000 \text{ units}}{\text{ml}} = \frac{750,000 \text{ units}}{x \text{ ml}}$$

    $$500,000x = 750,000$$

    $$x = 1.5 \text{ ml}$$

23. c. 16 oz = 480 ml

$$\frac{90 \text{ ml}}{480 \text{ ml}} = \frac{x \text{ ml}}{100 \text{ ml}}$$

$$480x = 9000$$

$$x = 18.75 \text{ ml}$$

If there are 18.75 ml of drug in 100 ml, the percentage is 18.75 or 18.8%.

24. c. $$\frac{69.12 \text{ gm}}{480 \text{ ml}} = \frac{x \text{ gm}}{100 \text{ ml}}$$

$$480x = 6912$$

$$x = 14.4 \text{ gm}$$

If there are 14.4 gm of drug in 100 ml, the percentage is 14.4%.

25. a. 120 ml/60 min × 10 gtt/ml = 20 gtt/min

26. b. 100 ÷ 15,000 = 0.00666 = 0.007%

27. c. 1 mg = 1000 mcg

10,000 mcg × 1 mg/1000 mcg = 10 mg

28. c. $$\frac{250,000 \text{ units}}{\text{ml}} = \frac{1,000,000 \text{ units}}{x \text{ ml}}$$

$$250,000x = 1,000,000$$

$$x = 4 \text{ ml}$$

29. c. $$\frac{5 \text{ mg}}{\text{ml}} = \frac{35 \text{ mg}}{x \text{ ml}}$$

$$5x = 35$$

$$x = 7 \text{ ml}$$

30. b.

20		10
	15	
5		5

Total

Parts 15

$$\frac{10}{15} \times 2000 \text{ ml} = 1333 \text{ ml of } 20\%$$

$$\frac{5}{15} \times 2000 \text{ ml} = 667 \text{ ml of } 5\%$$

Trade/Generic/Classification Practice Test I

1. c	2. d	3. a	4. c	5. b
6. c	7. b	8. b	9. d	10. c
11. d	12. b	13. a	14. d	15. d
16. b	17. b	18. c	19. b	20. d
21. b	22. d	23. c	24. b	25. c
26. c	27. d	28. d	29. a	30. b
31. b	32. b	33. d	34. d	35. b
36. c	37. a	38. c	39. c	40. a
41. c	42. c	43. b	44. c	45. d
46. b	47. c	48. c	49. d	50. d
51. d	52. b	53. c	54. d	55. d
56. b	57. c	58. b	59. c	60. d
61. a	62. c	63. d	64. d	65. d
66. b	67. b	68. a	69. c	70. b
71. b	72. b	73. c	74. d	75. a
76. c	77. c	78. b	79. b	80. c
81. b	82. c	83. a	84. d	85. a
86. b	87. d	88. a	89. d	90. b

Trade/Generic/Classification Practice Test II

1. c	2. a	3. c	4. b	5. a
6. b	7. c	8. b	9. a	10. b
11. c	12. b	13. b	14. b	15. a
16. b	17. d	18. d	19. d	20. c
21. c	22. c	23. b	24. b	25. c
26. c	27. b	28. c	29. a	30. a
31. c	32. a	33. b	34. c	35. d
36. a	37. d	38. a	39. a	40. d
41. a	42. b	43. d	44. a	45. b
46. c	47. b	48. a	49. a	50. d
51. b	52. c	53. d	54. b	55. a
56. d	57. b	58. a	59. b	60. c
61. a	62. a	63. c	64. c	65. c
66. a	67. d	68. c	69. b	70. c
71. c	72. a	73. a	74. c	75. b
76. c	77. d	78. d	79. d	80. b
81. d	82. a	83. b	84. d	85. b
86. b	87. a	88. c	89. a	90. b

Index